Treating Vulnerable Populations of Cancer Survivors: A Biopsychosocial Approach

Tanya R. Fitzpatrick
Editor

Treating Vulnerable Populations of Cancer Survivors: A Biopsychosocial Approach

Springer

Editor
Tanya R. Fitzpatrick
Department of Oncology
McGill University
Montreal
Canada

and

Department of Social Work
Arizona State University
Westmount
Canada

ISBN 978-3-319-32362-6 ISBN 978-3-319-32364-0 (eBook)
DOI 10.1007/978-3-319-32364-0

Library of Congress Control Number: 2016938396

Printed on acid-free paper

This Springer imprint is published by Springer Nature
The registered company is Springer International Publishing AG Switzerland

Contents

1 **Theoretical and Conceptual Models of Age and Ethnicity** 1
Tanya R. Fitzpatrick

2 **Providing Psychosocial Distress Screening, Coping Resources, and Self-care to Newly Diagnosed Cancer Survivors in a Canadian Small Town Setting** 7
Linda J. Edgar

3 **Latino Cancer Survivors: The Old and the Young** 23
Tanya R. Fitzpatrick

4 **An Exploration of Latvian Immigrants' Cancer Experience and Implications for Supportive Interventions** 37
Mara L. Leimanis

5 **Survivorship Issues Among Muslim Women with Cancer** 55
Suzanne Y. Bushfield

6 **Exploring the Artist's Book: How Art Therapy Can Benefit the Quality of Life of Young Adult Breast Cancer Survivors** 67
Katherine Laux

7 **Physical Activity, Locus of Control, and Fear of Recurrence Among Cancer Survivors from a Community-Based Cancer Support Program** 93
Roxana Mititelu, Achuthan Aruljothy and Tanya R. Fitzpatrick

8 **Oral Health Issues and Quality of Life Among Pediatric Cancer Survivors** 111
Crystal Noronha and Mary Ellen Macdonald

9 **Quality of Life Among Esophageal Cancer Survivors: Medical and Psychosocial Support** 127
Adriano Petrangelo, Mara L. Leimanis, Lorenzo Ferri and Tanya R. Fitzpatrick

10 The Family Caregiver as Cancer Survivor: Supporting and Promoting Positive Bereavement Outcomes 143
Lorraine Holtslander

Index 155

Editor and Contributors

About the Editor

Tanya R. Fitzpatrick, Ph.D., MSW, RN obtained her Ph.D. from Boston College Graduate School of Social Work and is Professor Emeritus from Arizona State University in Phoenix, Arizona (Department of Social Work) with a background in nursing, oncology, and gerontology. She was the Director of Research and Consultant at Hope & Cope in the Jewish General Hospital (2009–2013). More recently, she was a research consultant assisting on a project in the Department of Nursing at McGill University, Montreal. She is also mentoring first- and second-year McGill medical students in research projects focusing on cancer survivors and other health-related outcomes. Besides editing a book on ethnic elders, she has published more than 50 articles, book chapters in scientific journals, and received numerous grants.

Contributors

Achuthan Aruljothy, B.Sc. completed his undergraduate degree in Anatomy and Cell Biology from McGill University and continued to pursue his medical school training at McGill, where he is completing his final year. Working in numerous clinical settings throughout his medical education and having been involved in psychosocial research under the mentorship of Dr. Fitzpatrick has reinforced his goals and desires to practice primary care through a residency in internal medicine. He is a strong advocate of preventive care, patient education, and community outreach, which are fundamental to the art and science of medicine.

Suzanne Y. Bushfield, Ph.D., MSW (retired) after completing her Ph.D. she served as a Faculty Member and Researcher at Arizona State University, New Mexico State University, Lewis Clark State College, and the University of North Dakota. She ended her career as Accreditation Director for the Council of Social Work Education and as Chief Accreditation Operations Officer for the Association for the Accreditation of Human Research Protection Programs. Her research has focused on issues that have an impact on women's lives throughout the lifespan, including breast cancer and end-of-life caregiving.

Linda Edgar obtained her Ph.D. from McGill University, Montreal, Canada. Her research career focuses on psychosocial interventions for cancer patients and their families. She was instrumental in advocating for the use of the distress thermometer. She has published many referred articles and obtained grants from CIHR. She has held nursing positions as teacher, researcher, consultant, and clinician, and continues to stress the importance of good coping in all those roles.

Lorenzo Ferri, MD, Ph.D. FRCSC is Associate Professor of Surgery and Oncology at McGill University and Chief of Thoracic and Esophageal Surgery. As a thoracic surgeon, he has conducted and published numerous studies on the clinical outcomes of patients suffering from esophageal and lung cancer. In addition he runs the MUHC program in Upper GI Cancer, the largest and most comprehensive in Canada.

Lorraine Holtslander, RN, Ph.D., CHPCN(c) Honorary Associate Professor, University of the Witwatersrand, Johannesburg, South Africa is Associate Professor in the College of Nursing in Saskatoon, Canada with the University of Saskatchewan and a certified hospice palliative care nurse. Her clinical area is in Palliative Home Care, which supports the focus of her research in palliative care, specifically grief and loss, family caregiving and supporting family caregivers during bereavement.

Katherine Laux is art therapist (MA, ATPQ) and arts-based researcher in oncology at Cedars CanSupport, based at the McGill University Health Centre in Montreal, Québec. She is also affiliated with the Art Hive movement and offers an open art studio at La Ruche d'Art St-Henri for oncology patients and their loved ones. In addition to individual and group work, Kate organizes and co-curates public art exhibits of patient artwork. She also believes strongly in the healing aspects of art-making, and in the ability of supportive art-making sessions and group spaces to build connections and self-esteem, and to empower at any point of the cancer trajectory, including end-of-life care.

Mara L. Leimanis, Ph.D. with a background in biochemistry, has taken a special interest in translation research ("bench to bedside"), with over 7 years of experience in clinical research. In this time, she worked at the postdoctoral level abroad on the Thai–Burmese border with the migrant and refugee populations with the Mahidol-Oxford Research Unit based in Bangkok, Thailand. For the past 5 years, she has focused her research in medical and psychosocial oncology working in several hospitals in Montreal, Canada. Dr. Leimanis is a first-born generation Canadian-Latvian. She is now living in Grand Rapids, Michigan and is Senior Research Specialist with the Helen De Vos Childrens' Hospital.

Mary Ellen MacDonald, Ph.D. is Medical Anthropologist with postdoctoral training in Pediatric Palliative Care. She has an appointment in the Division of Oral Health and Society and is affiliated with the Departments of Pediatrics and Oncology, and the Ingram School of Nursing and Biomedical Ethics Unit. She is also Core Faculty in the McGill Centre for Medical Education. She chairs the McGill Qualitative Health Research group. Her main research interests include oral health in vulnerable populations, palliative care and bereavement, cultural aspects of health and illness with indigenous communities, and health professions education.

Roxana Mititelu, B.Sc. originally from Romania, completed a bachelor's of science at McGill and is now in her final year of medical school, also at McGill University. Roxana is passionate about complex medical care involving an interdisciplinary approach, so as to best provide whole-patient care. She has previously performed pre-clinical vaccine research and has a strong interest in oncology. She was a volunteer at the Hope & Cope Wellness Centre, at the Jewish General Hospital and later was hired as Research Assistant (2013–2014) working with Dr. Fitzpatrick on research projects focusing on cancer survivors.

Crystal Noronha, M.Sc. is Project Manager of the Views On Interdisciplinary Childhood Ethics (VOICE) project. She completed a graduate degree in dental sciences at McGill University, Montreal. She is currently working on scoping reviews on pediatric health and ethics and participates in studies addressing cancer survivors.

Adriano Petrangelo will obtain a Bachelor's degree in Anatomy and Cell Biology from McGill University (Spring, 2016). He worked as Research Assistant in the Department of Thoracic Surgery at the Montreal General Hospital in the lab of Dr. Lorenzo Ferri under the supervision of Dr. Mara Leimanis. His research has focused on esophageal cancer and medical and psychosocial outcomes. He worked on a project focusing on longitudinal HRQoL in esophageal cancer patients via patient-reported surveys throughout treatment at the Montreal General Hospital. He is a member of the McGill Varsity Baseball Team and hopes to pursue a career in medicine.

Introduction

The purpose of this book is to explore the relationships between a variety of therapeutic interventions and strategies as they impact the social and health issues among vulnerable populations of cancer survivors. Age and cultural behaviors are also examined as they relate to cancer survivors seeking community and hospital services. While research has been conducted on age and race, as it relates to mental and physical health outcomes among different ethnic groups, scant research has been directed towards appropriate interventions among vulnerable populations of cancer survivors.

The possibility of surviving cancer for longer periods of time is increasing with the likelihood of living with a challenging and chronic disease. Although cancer is primarily a disease of older adults, young adults and children from minority and ethnic groups experience different survival rates as compared to non-Hispanic Whites (Chao et al. 2014). Yet many ethnic populations continue to underutilize health and social services in spite of their higher level of need (Alemán et al. 2000). Ethnic minorities, especially the very young and elderly cancer survivors, are the underserved population creating a complex burden for oncology professionals and other health care workers—hence the need for this book. The necessity to understand survivorship issues from the onset of diagnosis is critical.

This book will provide further understanding for oncology professional and practitioners who must negotiate and provide optimum care for different ages and ethnic groups of cancer survivors during illness and recovery. Health care practitioners will need expertise in culturally competent practice to meet the needs and barriers that face cancer survivors and their family members.

The chapters in this book attempt to demonstrate the various challenges facing minority and different age groups with the goal of providing information on culturally appropriate strategies and interventions. Initially, though not exhaustive, theoretical and conceptual models are presented to help clarify the relationship between the different approaches and interventions and the quality of life among these populations.

Following this, Dr. Edgar begins by describing a pilot program that examines psychosocial outcomes such as distress, coping, and physical limitations, which are related to the delivery of psychosocial care to older cancer survivors living in a rural setting in Ontario, Canada. Many hospitals and clinics still struggle to find the best way to implement current interventions among the growing populations of older adults, and many oncology centers in Canada find it difficult to "buy-in" to the importance of psychosocial care. Detailed information on the demographics and history of psycho-oncology and the concept of cancer survivorship is also presented.

The next three chapters focus on the burden of cancer among ethnic minorities and how the use of various supportive resources and programs can make a more meaningful difference in their quality of life. For example, Dr. Fitzpatrick's chapter focuses on older and younger Latino cancer survivors and the use of various interventions such as leisure, household, and physical activities along with suggestions for the development of more appropriate community and supportive services. Development of therapeutic interventions has been problematic for Hispanic victims of cancer due to cultural barriers and demographic factors in determining health practices (Fitzpatrick and Farone 2011). Following this, Dr. Leimanis presents findings from her study investigating the effectiveness of family and community support among a group of Latvian cancer survivors residing in Montreal, Quebec. Her findings help to personalize the cancer experience of Latvians and the difficulties they face as immigrants and cancer survivors in a closed community such as privacy, isolation, language difficulties, and traditional norms. The next chapter by Dr. Bushfield attempts to address a neglected area in cancer research. Her study examines cancer survivorship issues among Muslim women living in America. Bushfield explores families that include a woman with cancer and how cultural beliefs, negative attention, and considerable discrimination have limited their access to timely health and social services.

Each of the following chapters highlights the special issues of both younger and older cancer survivors. Kate Laux's chapter explores how art therapy can benefit the quality of life among young breast cancer survivors. Younger women face fears of disfigurement and infertility, job- and family-related pressures along with changes associated with social relationships. Mititelu, Aruljothy, and Fitzpatrick examine the relationship between physical activities, locus of control, and the fear of cancer recurrence. Fear of cancer recurrence is a main concern negatively affecting the quality of life among cancer survivors despite psychosocial advances in treatment.

Following this, a chapter by Crystal Noronha and Mary Ellen MacDonald explores the impact on quality of life and therapy-related oral complications among pediatric cancer survivors. To date, dental care of pediatric cancer survivors is a neglected area. Her intention was to better understand the late effects of various cancer treatments and complications due to the interruption of therapy until tooth infections, caries, and abnormalities of the jaw can be resolved. Oral side effects of cancer therapy and related dental health problems impede social interaction and communication and are associated with pain, discomfort and problems with eating and sleeping.

Next, Petrangelo, Leimanis, Ferri and Fitzpatrick describe a study by providing the literature addressing psychosocial and medical issues among esophageal–gastric cancer survivors. Esophageal and gastric cancers are two of the most prevalent and devastating cancer diseases, especially for the elderly. Survivors face physical, psychological, social, and emotional distress due to the negative impact on clinical outcomes and survival. Little research to date has been undertaken to assess therapeutic interventions and the long-term effects of treatment on quality of life. Supportive programs in the community are scarce, however, the authors attempt to provide information on what is now available and offer suggestions for future programming and community services.

In conclusion, the final chapter by Dr. Holtslander captures the concept of the caregiver as "survivor" when caring for family members who have cancer. Although we have mainly focused on cancer survivors, family caregivers have suffered greatly and face many barriers during the process of attending to a loved one with cancer. The author provides new evidence for caregiver support initiatives that include comprehensive assessment and person-centered approaches to address the specific needs and burdens of the caregiver survivor, also focusing on the interaction between the needs of the caregiver and the family member with cancer.

Although cancer survivors from all walks of life are confronted with emotional and physical challenges on a daily basis, each of the chapters in this book highlight the added barriers that survivors from several different ethnic and age groups experience. In summary, this book will illustrate the most current thinking into the design and delivery of therapeutic interventions addressing the needs of several vulnerable groups of cancer survivors and how oncology professionals and practitioners may be better informed to practice more effectively.

Demographics

Despite scientific gains over the last 10 years, many ethnic minorities and other underserved populations experience higher cancer incidence and mortality rates than the general population (U.S. Cancer Statistics 2014). The diagnosis of cancer is clearly a health-related problem for everyone, regardless of age or ethnicity (Fitzpatrick and Farone 2011).

Pediatric Cancer Survivors

In Canada alone, childhood cancer is the second leading case of death in children under the age of 14 (Noronha 2012, Masters Thesis in Dental Sciences). However, survival rates have increased (83 %) due to aggressive cancer treatments (Canadian Cancer Society 2014; Erickson and Steiner 2001). The main types of childhood cancers are leukemia, brain and central nervous system tumors, lymphomas, sarcomas, and liver and kidney cancers, with leukemia being the most common type (Noronha 2012). Leukemia accounts for 33 % of childhood cancers in Canada. Noronha explains that childhood cancers quite often occur as a result of changes in cells before birth, yet are said to have a better survival rate than many adults cancer; however, the side effects may be greater. Many of the treatments for these types of cancers affect the oral cavity of the child and oral side effects may occur during or soon after treatment and can also exist months after remission. The impact on the quality of life and survivorship can be both traumatic and challenging for the child and their family members.

Adolescents and Young Adult Survivors (AYAs)
Adolescents and young adults, from age 15 to 39 years, have fared less well and have not experienced the same degree of survival rates as younger and older adults (Bleyer et al. 2006; Chao et al. 2014). This is the result of lack of attention from cancer professionals, few national clinical trials, and or limited access to optimal cancer services. This group has been "caught between two worlds" and should now be seen as a distinct age group (Bleyer et al. 2006, p. 1645). In the U.S. cancer is the leading cause of death (non-accidental) among adolescents and young adults. Bleyer et al. (2006) describe two age groups of survivors: older adolescents aged 15–19 years and young adults aged 20–39 years. The impact on the 15–19 year olds is far greater as their health care needs are adversely affected. There are fewer young adults able to enter the job market due to health-related treatment, plus they experience the social implications of cancer during early adulthood. Adolescents in this group also have unique medical and psychosocial needs as the biology of their malignancies are unique.

The Elderly Cancer Survivor
By 2050, 21 % of older adults will be 80 years and older. Cancer is the leading cause of death among both men and women over the age of 60. "Cancer is primarily a disease of older adults " (Surbone et al. 2007, p. 633). Alemán et al. (2000) report that ethnic elders who have been disenfranchised will be in greater need to receive services because of the increased number of elders, especially those with cancer. Although the survival rates for cancer are increasing due to early detection and advanced treatment interventions, the quality of one's health becomes an ongoing challenge for health care professionals, family members, and cancer survivors. Older cancer survivors in particular may experience "the detrimental effects of a cancer diagnosis in addition to age-related chronic diseases and chronic limitations" (Fitzpatrick et al. 2012, p. 567). However, the diagnosis of cancer is clearly a health problem regardless of age or ethnicity (Fitzpatrick and Farone 2011).

Tanya R. Fitzpatrick

References

Alemán, S., Fitzpatrick, T. R., Tran, T. V., & Gonzalus, E. (Eds.). (2000). *Therapeutic interventions with ethnic elders: Health and social issues.* New York, London: The Hayworth Press.

Bleyer, A., Budd' T., & Montello, M. (2006). Adolescents and young adults with cancer. The scope of the problem and criticality of clinical trials. *Cancer, 107* (7 Suppl), 1645–1655. doi:10.1002/cncr. 22102.

Canadian Cancer Society. (2014). Canadian Cancer Statistics Publication. (2015). *In Canadian Cancer Society*. Info@cis.cancer.ca.

Chao, C., Chiu, V. Y., Xu, L., & Cooper, R. M. (2014). Survival differences by *race/ethnicity in adolescents and young adults diagnosed with non-Hodgkin*.lymphoma. Poster Presentation: The ASCO Annual Meeting. (2014). Published on *Meeting Library*. http://meetinglibrary.asco.org.

Erickson, S., & Steiner, H. (2001). Trauma and personality correlates in long-term pediatric cancer survivors. *Child Psychiatry & Human Development, 31,* 195–213.

Farone, D. W., Fitzpatrick, T. R., & Bushfield, S. Y. (2008). Hope, locus of control, and quality of health among elder Latina cancer survivors. *Social Work in Healthcare, 46*, 51–70.

Fitzpatrick, T. R., & Farone, D. W. (2011). Leisure, household activities and health among Mexican American elders with cancer. *Journal of Psychosocial Oncology, 29,* 199–214.

Fitzpatrick, T. R., Edgar, L., & Holcroft, C. (2012). Assessing the relationship between physical fitness activities, cognitive health and quality of life among older cancer survivors. *Journal of Psychosocial Psychology, 30*, 556–572.

Noronha, C. (2012). Impact on quality of life due to therapy-related oral complications in pediatric cancer patients: A scoping review. *M.Sc. Manuscript based*, Montreal, Canada: McGill University.

Surbone, A., Kagawa-Singer, M., Terret, C., & Baider, L. (2007). The illness trajectory of elderly cancer patients across cultures: SIOG position paper. *Annuals of Oncology, 18*, 633–638.

U.S. Cancer Statistics. (2014). *In CA Cancer/Clin 2014 64*, 9–29. onlinelibrary.wiley.com/doi/10.3322/caac.21208/pdf

Chapter 1
Theoretical and Conceptual Models of Age and Ethnicity

Tanya R. Fitzpatrick

This chapter will provide an overview of various theoretical and conceptual models in an attempt to clarify the relationships between a variety of therapeutic interventions that address social and health issues among vulnerable populations of cancer survivors. These theories also assist in understanding the challenges different age and ethnic groups face when living with a life threatening disease such as cancer. Although some theories have addressed older adults from different ethnic age groups, few theories have addressed the barriers and challenges that young children and young adult cancer survivors face in society today.

Cancer-Related Quality of Life

Quality of life (QOL) is defined as a broad multidimensional construct that includes emotional, social, sexual, cognitive, and physical functioning as perceived by the individual (Yanez et al. 2011). The concept of cancer-related QOL is discussed in more detail in many of the following chapters. It is associated with all aspects of cancer survival and interventions that address physical and mental health outcomes.

Stress and Coping Mechanism

The suffering that has been attributed to a diagnosis of cancer and survival can be examined through the conceptual framework of the stress and coping mechanism and the process and ability of the individual to adapt to a usually fatal disease such as

T.R. Fitzpatrick (✉)
Department of Social Work, Arizona State University, 449 Mount Pleasant Ave., Westmount, QC H3Y3G9, Canada
e-mail: tanya.fitzpatrick@asu.edu

T.R. Fitzpatrick (ed.), *Treating Vulnerable Populations of Cancer Survivors: A Biopsychosocial Approach*, DOI 10.1007/978-3-319-32364-0_1

cancer (Barroilhet Diez et al. 2005). This model explains the influence of adaptation to cancer including sociocultural, psychological, and medical factors. The stress process begins when the individual realizes that there is no escape from the diagnosis of cancer. Fear and confusion may result from the uncertainty of the present and future health status. Coping is defined as "the specific thoughts and behaviors that a person uses in his/her efforts to adapt to the cancer" (Folkman and Greer 2000, p. 11). However, coping strategies are not always effective in controlling the distress associated with the changes that occur emotionally, socially, and with medical treatment during the individual's life circumstances. (See Barroilhet Diez et al. 2005, for a detailed description of the stress and coping process as it relates to cancer.)

Ethnicity and Aging

Although, a number of theories of aging have attempted to address ethnic elders and various mental and physical health outcomes, limited investigations have focused on ethnic elders with cancer (Alemán et al. 2000). There are several popular models and theories that focus on ethnicity and aging such as the *double jeopardy hypothesis* (Butler et al. 1991; Dowd and Bengston 1978), *modernization theory* (Cowgill and Holmes 1972; Markides and Mindel 1987), *assimilation theory* (Markides and Mindel 1987), and *acculturation* and *cultural pluralism* (Healey 1996; Fitzpatrick 2000; Tran et al. 1996). There are also more recent investigations such as ethnic "homogeneity and otherness," (Zubair and Victor 2014). They state that these frameworks perceive and position older people in essentialist terms by focusing upon and over-empathizing their ethnic and older age "difference" and vulnerability. (See Zubair and Norris 2015, for a complete review of perspectives and theories of aging and ethnicity.) Yet these current models do not address ethnic elders with cancer. Regardless, this body of literature provides a basic understanding of how culture and ethnicity is particularly important when providing services to elders of color and the diversity of experiences between and within the various groups.

Perspectives on Aging, Culture, and Cancer

The concept of "*mastery*", which is described as one's "perceived control over circumstances," (Surbone et al. 2007, p. 636) and "*self-efficacy*," defined as one's ability to accomplish tasks and address age appropriate responsibilities and goals, represent two important themes that address an older adult's ability to adjust and cope with a diagnosis of cancer. Factors such as age, gender, culture, living arrangements, available family, and community supports will also influence the manner in which an older person adjusts and copes with cancer. Surbone et al. (2007) report that culture and the individual's response to a life threatening illness in particular are shaped by his or her view of the world.

The "*strength-based perspective*", which is rooted in empowerment theory (Blondo 2001; Graybeal 2001), is based on the concept of self-determination, and can in turn lead to successful and positive mental health outcomes among those with life threatening illnesses such as cancer (Farone et al. 2008). The concept of *hope and locus of control* as described by Farone et al. (2008), suggests that "cognitive structural expectations affect behavior and emotional states," (Farone et al. 2008, p. 54; Wallston et al. 1994). Specifically related to elderly individuals with cancer, a strong internal locus of control is associated with better adjustment to cancer (Watson et al. 1990), yet some studies of locus of control and psychological outcomes have mixed results, in that no or little association was found between locus of control and prognosis for cancer (Garssen 2004). Some studies also lend support to the positive influence from having a strong internal locus of control as experienced with some health and well-being outcomes. Therefore, the findings of associations between the concept of internal locus of control and quality of health especially for elderly Latino cancer survivors (Farone et al. 2008) suggest that interventions should address and attempt to strengthen personal and individual coping resources. Interventions that are designed to foster hope may produce positive changes on quality of live among cancer survivors regardless of age or ethnicity (Baker et al. 1994; Farone et al. 2008).

Theoretical Perspectives as a Guide to Interventions with Pediatric and Adolescent Cancer Survivors

As well as other severe traumatic changes and losses, *posttraumatic stress disorder* (PTSD) has been applied to the understanding of cancer-related responses among childhood cancer survivors (Bruce 2006; Erickson and Steiner 2001; Stuber et al. 1997). Over time, the child can be exposed to extreme stress during the diagnosis, treatment, and remission phase of the disease resulting in dissociation, somatization, and dysregulation. The symptoms of posttraumatic stress are described by Erickson and Steiner (2001) as: (1) reexperiencing the traumatic event, (2) persistent avoidance of circumstances and reminders of the traumatic event, and (3) anxiety, avoidance, and concentration difficulties along with intrusive memories (Stuber et al. 1997). These authors report that the predictors of PSTD symptoms in children and adolescence are factors related to anxiety and subjective appraisal rather than from the actual treatment of the disease. In some cases symptoms may decrease over time, yet for others, even after five years of posttreatment, high levels of PTSD reflect the long-term negative effects of childhood cancer for both the survivors and their family members.

Other theories have attempted to focus on positive health rather than pathology models in psychosocial adjustment among adolescent cancer survivors. Haase (2004) emphasizes the fact that the concept of "*resilience*" or the adolescent resilience model (ARM) is a guide to effective interventions as the notion of hope, positive coping, and social support contribute to a positive outcome and the improvement of QOL for this age group (Haase 2004). The *resilience model* has recently been applied to veterans and their informal caregivers (Smith-Osbourne and Felderhoff 2014) as an intervention model for oncologists and social work practitioners specifically focusing on active-duty service members and for military families in pre- and post-deployment stages. Resilience is defined as "relative resistance to adversity or risk" (p. 557). As adolescent cancer survivors are a neglected group in the area of receiving psychosocial services and interventions, the resilience model offers some understanding and hope that supports can address the specific physical and emotional needs leading to a more positive adjustment to their cancer experience (Haase 2004). Resilience-based strategies not only target the child or adolescent but the family as a unit, which might include the need for leisure, recreation, spirituality, peer relationships, identity formation along with continued support, and community referrals from health care professionals (Haase 2004).

Finally, the *culture and social class* model as described by Marshall et al. (2011) attempts to bring together the experience of cancer for the individual and their family members by advancing a model of health promotion and psychosocial interventions that acknowledges the understanding of social class. The social class of an individual can present barriers to available interventions, as culture and social class are thus essential for our understanding of the family members' response to cancer. Existing theories and frameworks have primarily focused on white and middle class families and have neglected to include those from low income and ethnically diverse populations. Family systems and sociocultural frameworks propose that social class, culture, values, beliefs, language, and family customs are important factors for health care professionals to address. How the individual and their family members, especially underserved populations, respond to the challenging diagnosis of cancer leading to successful therapeutic interventions is needed more now than ever. The health and well-being of the individual with cancer and their family depends on community-based supports that address not only their medical needs but psychosocial and social class issues as well (Marshall et al. 2011; Smith-Osbourne and Felderhoff 2014).

References

Alemán, S., Fitzpatrick, T. R., Tran, T. V., & Gonzalus, E. (Eds.). (2000). *Therapeutic interventions with ethnic elders: Health and social issues*. New York, London: The Hayworth Press.

Baker, L. A., Cesa, I. L., Gatz, M., & Mellins, C. (1994). Genetic and environmental influences on positive and negative affect. *Psychology and Aging, 7*, 158–163.

Barroilhet Diez, S., Foriaz, M. J., & Garrido Landivar, E. (2005). Concepts, theories and psychosocial factors in cancer adaption. *Actas Esp Psiquiatr, 33*, 390–397.

Blondo, R. (2001). Learning strength-based practice: Challenging our personal and Professional frames. *Families in Society, 82*, 296–304.

Bruce, M. (2006). A systematic and conceptual review of posttraumatic stress in childhood cancer survivors and their parents. *Clinical Psychology Review, 26*, 233–256.

Butler, R. N., Lewis, M., & Sunderland, T. (1991). *Aging and mental health: Positive psychosocial and biomedical approaches*. New York: Macmillan Publishing Company.

Cowgill, D. O., & Holmes, L. (1972). *Aging and modernization*. New York: Appleton-Century-Crofts.

Dowd, J. J., & Bengston, V. (1978). Aging in minority populations: An examination of the double jeopardy hypothesis. *Journal of Gerontology, 33*, 427–436.

Erickson, S., & Steiner, H. (2001). Trauma and personality correlates in long-term pediatric cancer survivors. *Child Psychiatry and Human Development, 31*, 195–213.

Farone, D. W., Fitzpatrick, T. R., & Bushfield, S. Y. (2008). Hope, locus of control, and quality of health among elder Latina cancer survivors. *Social Work in Health Care, 46*, 51–70.

Fitzpatrick, T. R. (2000). Elderly Russian Jewish immigrants. In S. Alemán, T. R. Fitzpatrick, T. V. Tran, & E. Gonzalus (Eds.), *Therapeutic interventions with ethnic elders: Health and social issues*. New York, London: The Hayworth Press.

Folkman, S., & Greer, S. (2000). Promoting psychosocial well-being in the face of serious Illness: When theory, research and practice inform each other. *Psycho-Oncology, 9*, 11–19.

Garssen, B. (2004). Psychological factors and cancer development: Evidence after 30 years of research. *Clinical Psychology Review, 24*, 315–338.

Graybeal, C. (2001). Strengths-based social work assessment: Transforming the dominant Paradigm. *Families in Society, 82*, 233–242.

Haase, J. E. (2004). The adolescent resilience model as a guide to interventions. *Journal of Pediatric Nursing, 21*, 289–299.

Healey, J. F. (1996). *Race, ethnicity and gender in the U.S.* Thousand Oaks, CA: Pine Forge Press.

Markides, K. S., & Mindel, C. H. (1987). *Aging and ethnicity*. Newbury Park, CA: Sage Publications.

Marshall, C. A., Larkey, L. K., Curran, M. A., Weihs, K. L., Badger, T. A., Armin, J., et al. (2011). Considerations of culture and social class for families facing cancer: The need for a new model fro health promotion and psychosocial intervention. *Family Systems Health, 29*, 81–94.

Smith-Osbourne, A., & Felderhoff, B. (2014). Veterans' informal caregivers in the "sandwich generation": A systematic review toward a resilience model. *Journal of Gerontological Social Work, 57*, 556–573.

Stuber, M. L., Kazek, A. E., Meeske, K., Baraket, L., Guthrie, D., Garnier, H., et al. (1997). Predictors of posttraumatic stress symptoms in childhood cancer survivors. *Pediatrics, 100*, 958–964.

Surbone, A., Kagawa-Singer, M., Terret, C., & Baider, L. (2007). The illness trajectory of elderly cancer patients across cultures: SIOG position paper. *Annuals of Oncology, 18*, 633–638.

Tran, T. V., Fitzpatrick, T. R., Berg, W. R., & Wright, R, Jr. (1996). Acculturation, health, stress and psychological distress among elderly Hispanics. *Journal of Cross-Cultural Gerontology, 11*, 149–165.

Wallston, K. A., Stein, M. J., & Smith, C. A. (1994). Form C of the MHLC scales: A condition-specific measure of locus of control. *Journal of Personality Assessment, 38*, 534–553.

Watson, M., Pruyn, J., Greer, S., & Van den Borne, B. (1990). Locus of control and adjustment to cancer. *Psychological Reports, 66*, 39–48.

Yanez, B., Thompson, E. H., & Stanton, A. L. (2011). Quality of life among Latina breast cancer patients: A systematic review of the literature. *Journal of Cancer Survivorship, 5*(2), 191–207. doi:10.1007/s11764-011-0171-0. Epub 2011 Jan 28.

Zubair, M., & Norris, M. (2015). Perspectives on aging, later life, and ethnicity: Aging research in ethnic minority contexts. *Aging Society, 35*(5), 897–916. doi:10.1017/S0144

Zubair, M., & Victor, C. (2014). Marginalizing research "ethics": Issues of "othering:" Resistance and (dis) empowerment in research involving other ethnic minority people. Paper presented at the British Society of Gerontology, Scotland seminar *Marginalization in later life*, November 5, University of the West of Scotland, UK.

Chapter 2
Providing Psychosocial Distress Screening, Coping Resources, and Self-care to Newly Diagnosed Cancer Survivors in a Canadian Small Town Setting

Linda J. Edgar

Introduction and Background

Over 12 million new cases of cancer are diagnosed worldwide every year. This number is projected to increase to about 19 million by 2024 and double by 2050. As a result of improved treatments and knowledge there are now over 28 million survivors living with a personal history of cancer. While most survivors adjust well over the long term, others do not and few receive comprehensive care that meets their needs. In many ways, the race to find more effective bio-medical treatments appears to have outpaced the search for ways to aid patients' psychosocial well-being.

Psycho-oncology is the specialty that studies the psychological, social, and spiritual factors that affect the quality of life of cancer patients and their loved ones. Psycho-oncology contributes to the multidisciplinary approach to cancer through its role in clinical care, education, and research. Because of the formation of psycho-oncology as a discipline, guidelines and standards for psychosocial care have been developed and endorsed by several national and international scientific societies.

Cancer rehabilitation and survivorship care focus on rebuilding the lives of those with cancer and maximizing functioning and quality of life. Many care plans begin as treatment ends to prepare patients for their return to a new normal phase of life. These plans are meant to empower and inform both the survivor and the health-care team. There are fewer care plans for newly diagnosed patients, although research has shown that early intervention for distress can enhance compliance and efficacy of treatment, reduce side effects, and improve quality of life and satisfaction. As the

L.J. Edgar (✉)
Department of Nursing, Brock University, St. Catharines, ON, Canada
e-mail: lindajeanedgar@gmail.com

T.R. Fitzpatrick (ed.), *Treating Vulnerable Populations of Cancer Survivors: A Biopsychosocial Approach*, DOI 10.1007/978-3-319-32364-0_2

Institutes of Medicine (IOM, US) stated, "some elements of care simply make sense to improve patients' experience of living with cancer" (Vos et al. 2015).

Thus, the statement, "no health without mental health" has become the basis of standards and clinical guidelines for cancer care in many countries around the world including Canada. According to the National Cancer Institute's *Dictionary of Cancer Terms* (2012), the concept of cancer survivorship encompasses:

The physical, psychosocial, and economic issues of cancer exist from diagnosis until the end of life. These issues focus on the health and life of a person with cancer beyond the diagnosis and treatment phases [and] include issues related to the ability to get health care and follow-up treatment, late effects of treatment, second cancers, and quality of life. Over the last 25 years, many studies in psychosocial oncology have found that 30–40 % of cancer patients have difficulty in adapting, and have emotional disorders, such as depression, anxiety, irritable mood, and feelings of demoralization (Meyer and Mark 1995). Clinically significant distress is linked to reduction in well-being, quality of life, poor adherence to treatment, and a longer time to recover. Caregivers are also not immune to such distress, which is linked to their own psychosocial morbidity (Sundar et al. 2013).

Prevention of distress is a proactive position that provides patients with coping skills and resource tools, thus making them able to successfully handle their cancer journey. Patients, survivors, caregivers, and health-care personnel in Canada have long been advocating for a total care person-centered cancer system—one that intentionally focuses on what is of importance to the patient and attends to the range of his or her needs (not just the tumor). They require quality care that is comprehensive, coordinated, and continuous. They want future patients to have a better experience during the cancer journey than the current system provides. In such an improved scenario, the inter-professional team works in partnership with the cancer patient and his or her family to ensure that care is responsive, person-centered, and tailored to their specific needs. In recent years, three significant events have occurred in Canada to spearhead the move to person-centered oncology care: First, The Cancer Control Strategy for Canada has mandated that all patients be screened for distress starting at diagnosis, using standardized recommended measures, and referring those with distress to community or hospital resources. A recent set of guidelines for screening and assessment and care of psychosocial distress in Canada has advocated specific actions for all adult cancer patients. Second, providing psychosocial care to cancer patients is now an accreditation standard with the Canadian Hospital Accreditation Board for Regional Cancer Centers. Third, distress is now considered to be the sixth vital sign in caring for hospitalized and community-based patients, (following the five vital signs of temperature, pulse, respirations, blood pressure, and level of pain (Bultz and Johansen 2011).

A substantial number of peer-reviewed meta analytic research studies have tested various psychosocial educational interventions delivered by professionals or volunteers, and concluded that patients benefited from positive outcomes. Research has shown that early intervention for distress enhances compliance and efficacy of treatment, reduces side effects, and improves quality of life and satisfaction. A systematic review involving breast cancer patients found that positive coping strategies and a confident self-appraisal of the threat of the disease were among the most frequently reported factors linked to post-traumatic growth (Andersen et al. 2008). In another study, coping well during treatment and feeling a sense of personal control were found to mediate the relationship between physical symptoms and depression when treatment is over (Jacobsen 2009). Patients receiving radiotherapy who had a sense of self-efficacy before treatment had less symptom severity and anxiety post-treatment (Jacobsen et al. 2011). Lowering stress mediated the relationship between stress management skills and both physical functioning and emotional well-being for advanced prostate cancer survivors (Giesler et al. 2005).

Fostering patients' self-management has frequently been an area of relative weakness (Coleman and Newton 2005; Fitch 2009; Whitney et al. 2015). Most cancer patients are not currently adopting healthy behaviors, such as exercise and good nutrition, a fact which ultimately results in greater disease risks and health-care costs (Grant et al. 2012). Self-care strategies are not only useful in the transition to post-treatment care, but they are also useful in the diagnostic and early treatment phase to manage the ongoing effects of treatment. Active patient engagement plans empower and help return a sense of personal control, as their role in recovery becomes evident. Such plans are considered components of person-centered care where the needs of each individual are taken into account (Stanton 2012).

Many programs continue to rely on a group counseling model with supplemental written or internet-based information (Spiegel et al. 2007). We know that patients' preferences for the type of support they receive is the strongest predictor of a programs' success (Whitney et al. 2015). Several models have been proposed to meet the needs of cancer patients; however the shared-care approach has generally been accepted as the optimal way to meet those needs (Carlson et al. 2004). An essential component of any model is to share relevant patient information among the various health-care professionals involved in a timely manner.

In spite of the enormous work carried out by the founders of psych-oncology, such as Dr. Jimmie Holland, many hospitals and clinics still struggle to find the best way to implement current recommendations. There has been an increase in person-centered care, but screening and intervening are costly in both time and money. One step that has been somewhat neglected involves the development of an action-oriented self-care patient and family introduction to screening with appropriate follow-up steps. While most cancer centers recognize the value of having a program for newly diagnosed patients, they also want to design their own programs to fit with their beliefs and resources. Busy oncology centers, even in Canada, find it difficult to achieve a true "buy-in" to the importance of psychosocial care. We were interested in developing a simple platform that could be easily adopted and modified by individual centers into their own personalized programs. Pre-empting problems that may arise is a form of prerehabilitation that has been advocated (Silver and Baima 2013). We have noted that survivorship care plans can increase patients' feelings of confidence, satisfaction, and well-being; could a plan based on engaging patients in self-care strategies presented at the start of treatment be feasible and produce positive results? (Lauver et al. 2007; Silver and Baima 2013).

This chapter presents a pilot program to address current issues of time, personnel, process, content, and outcomes related to the delivery of psychosocial care to newly diagnosed middle aged or older adults living in a primarily rural setting in Ontario, Canada. This project was not a research study but the pilot implementation of a simple screening and patient education plan. Our goal was to develop a brief, one-time session working with individual patients and a significant family member using self-care strategies that would lower their levels of distress. The program was designed to screen newly diagnosed patients for distress, educate them on how to monitor themselves for distress, and seek out appropriate resources. To further empower patients and their families, we presented a brief introduction to basic coping strategies (Edgar 2010).

Intervention

We based the program on the constructs of coping appraisal and efficacy. When confronted by a diagnosis of cancer, people typically engage in the cognitive process of appraising the nature of the stressor (e.g., threat, actual harm, or loss) and whether they have the means to cope with it. Coping appraisal of one's cancer has been related to anxiety and adjustment in that the higher the perceived threat, the lower the level of well-being and the greater the level of distress (Lazarus and Folkman 1984). Coping efficacy is a form of self-efficacy that refers to people's beliefs about their ability to negotiate particular stressors or obstacles. These beliefs are assumed to affect how people perceive and react to adverse life events and conditions. Favorable perceptions of coping efficacy are likely to help people organize and deploy the coping methods at their disposal, draw effectively on environmental supports, and persist at problem solving when faced with difficult conditions. In the domain of cancer survivorship, coping efficacy includes beliefs about one's ability to deal with myriad challenges posed by the cancer experience, such as coping with treatment-related side effects, seeking and understanding medical information, and obtaining support to manage treatment and recovery. Although the literature on cancer-specific coping efficacy is somewhat limited at this point, available data suggest that stronger efficacy is related to positive outcomes such as higher quality of life (QOL) and fewer negative emotions (Lauver et al. 2007; Silver and Baima 2013).

The session was introduced to staff and patients as a step in the development of total patient care with the emphasis on meeting the psychosocial and educational needs of the person with cancer and his or her family. At the start of the session, for evaluative purposes, the following screening and assessment tools were administered as paper and pencil forms:

1. *The Edmonton Symptom Assessment Scale* (*ESAS*) (Bruera et al. 1991).
   ESAS assesses nine symptoms that are common to most cancer patients: pain, tiredness, nausea, depression, anxiety, drowsiness, appetite, well-being, and

shortness of breath. The severity of each symptom on a rating scale of 0–10 is measured by the patient at the time of the assessment. It is the patient's perception of the severity of the symptom that matters.

2. *The Canadian Problem checklist* (3).
   This is a short list of problems in six domains; practical, emotional, physical, spiritual, social, and informational. These items have been reported in peer-reviewed literature to be correlates of distress.
3. *The Distress Thermometer*
   On a scale of 1–10 where 0 means no distress at all and 10 refers to the worst distress possible, patients recorded where they stood at a designated time period such as the present moment or day (Bultz and Johansen 2011). Box 1 illustrates the Distress Thermometer.

Box 1: The Distress Thermometer

Learning to measure and manage your stress can make a difference in your life. In fact, in health care today distress (or stress) is now known as the sixth vital sign (after temperature, pulse, respirations, blood pressure, and pain). The best way to keep your distress in check and to know that you are still in control of your life is to cope well.

The Distress Thermometer is a simple tool that lets you measure your distress, take charge of it, and helps identify what is causing it. Continue to measure your distress , and follow the recommendations for your score.

How to use the Distress Thermometer

Circle the number that best describes the distress you have felt in the past week. Next, check the boxes on the Canadian Problem List that apply to you to identify what has been contributing to your distress. Find resources as needed to help deal with your concerns.

We followed the recommendations provided by the Pan Canadian Practice Guidelines developed by expert panelists and a critical literature review carried out by members of the Canadian Partnership against Cancer, and the Canadian Association of Psychosocial Oncology (CAPO) for screening, assessment, and appropriate referral to community or hospital resources. The distress algorithms were guidelines to appropriate referrals according to the patient's level of distress. The facilitators for this pilot program were the author and an experienced social worker/family counselor. We met individually with patients and a family member of their choice within 6 weeks of their first appointment with the oncology team. Each session lasted an average of 45 min. The format for the session has been operationalized and standardized for teaching and implementation, primarily through close adherence to the content and order of the booklet.

The facilitators began by stressing the values of learning to cope well, regaining a sense of personal control, and keeping track of distress levels that could interfere with good health and well-being. We provided a booklet on coping, developed initially by the West London Cancer Network, UK, and adapted and renamed, *Cancer Coping Resource Program, Coping with distress: Making a difference.* The contents included the distress thermometer with instructions, the Canadian Problem list, resources specific to individual needs, and several coping strategies. The booklet was divided into two sections, one which provided specific support services, resources, and useful contacts in the local area, and other explained the importance of screening for distress and ways of preventing its severity through active participation in one's health care and learning coping strategies that took advantage of each patient's individual strengths (Miaskowski 2004). Boxes 2 and 3 provide further excerpts from the booklet.

Box 2: Booklet Introduction

Having cancer is like taking a car trip over a hazardous road with oil spills, accidents, bumps, and very hot weather. How do you prepare for such a journey? You set some goals at the start. You intend to keep a helpful, hopeful, and realistic attitude whether your journey goes smoothly or not. You expect to have a good trip while being ready for any setbacks. For example, you anticipate comfort and safety with air conditioning, seatbelts, and air bags, and you also prepare for troubles by bringing extra oil, water, and spare tires with you.

Your goal for your cancer journey is to travel your route with a sense of personal control, having a healthy body and following your treatment plan. Coping well with whatever happens means you will experience a more successful journey.

Here are three "doable" objectives for us to work on today so that you can continue with them at home:

1. Become an active participant in your own care and life.
2. Realize that you can handle whatever comes your way because you have both inner strength and available resources.
3. Measure your distress level and keep it low through good coping.

When you are on your journey and when you look back on it, you want to be able to say that you handled it well. We do not have control over what happens to us, but we have total control over how we cope with it, and that makes all the difference.

What is good coping?

It is a active problem solving that is optimistic, flexible, realistic, and practical, and lifts you beyond distress and despair. It is having a plan to look after yourself to achieve a calm sense of personal control. Coping well is linked to a better cancer journey.

A goal needs a plan or else it is merely a wish, so here is a simple, workable plan to achieve good coping and lower distress.

- Complete the distress thermometer and the problem list on the following pages.
- Practice some good ways of coping.
- Find and use resources that are helpful and meet your needs.

Box 3: Excerpt from booklet on tools for coping

Some Good Coping Tools

Exercise of some kind 5 days out of 7, and keeping active in general are more than suggestions, they are essential to your well-being. Even small amounts of exercise a few minutes at a time are better than nothing, so feel good about starting small. Getting in better physical shape is a goal for you. What are your plans for doing it?

Remember how you successfully coped with stressful times in the past. Think about some of the things you are doing now to help you cope, for example; talking to close friends and family, going out, exercising, listening to music, and keeping a hopeful frame of mind. Identifying your strengths, and patting yourself on the back for them, can help you understand and be grateful for them.

List some of your strengths that have helped you cope well throughout your life:

____

Learn to deal with a changed health-care system

The biggest change in today's health-care system is a shift from the patient being passive to being an active member of the team. You are the expert on your own body and yourself. Take ownership for making your body as healthy as possible—through eating well, having a good balance between exercise, rest and sleep, and coping with stress. Exercise is especially effective at reducing pain, fatigue, and improving mood and sleep.

You are the center of your health-care team. It is up to you to express yourself, say what is important to you and ask questions. Be as much a part of decision-making about your care as you want. When patients participate in their fight for recovery they move from feeling helpless to feeling in control.

Before your doctor's appointment, write down any concerns and questions so you do not forget to ask them, and ask for simple explanations to make sure you understand. Take someone with you to be another pair of ears and eyes. Having a friend or relative support you is important to your well-being. Medical care today is complicated and needs lots of coordination among many people who are doing the best they can. No news or information about your care may mean that somehow something has been forgotten or slipped through the cracks. If in doubt, ask!

Other tools included in the booklet

Learn how your thoughts affect your feelings.

Deep breathing

Mindful meditation

In summary, you now can measure your level of stress and have six proven coping tools to practice. We know these will make your cancer journey easier and healthier. You will have done your best, and will feel that sense of personal control.

Patients were not asked to give a history of their treatments or illness, but simply to recount their most pertinent issues using the ESAS and the problem list. The facilitators did not have access to patients' medical records, and the only information required was the name of their oncologist and the patients' birth date, for purposes of identification and transfer of summary information. Our intentions were to educate them about their role in managing their health and well-being and show them how to measure and handle their distress at home through the use of resources and coping strategies. In particular, the session emphasized the value of exercise, the need to regain a sense of personal control, be aware of one's own strengths, and take an active role in health care. Mindful meditation, deep breathing, and a schematic of how thoughts influence feelings were also presented.

A specific plan for future distress management was designed in collaboration with each patient. After the session was over, the facilitators completed a brief summary page on the patient's status, which was forwarded to the treating team. (Refer to Box 4).

Box 4: Results from the Oncology Distress Management Program

Name of Patient ______________________ Date____________

Total ESAS score________________

Pain____ Tired____ Nausea____ Depression____ Anxiety____
Drowsy____ Appetite_____ Wellbeing____ Dyspnea_____

Distress Thermometer Level___________

Canadian Problem List ___________

Practical

Emotional

Physical

Spiritual

Social

Informational

Resources given

Comments

Two month follow up

Date scheduled

Outcome

CopeSmart Signature

Oncology Clinic Review Signature

We telephoned patients up to 2 months later to reassess their distress level and provide resources as needed. Two university nursing students were hired to carry out the final evaluation by phone between 3 and 4 months, using Likert scales and open-ended questions.

Results

There were 612 newly diagnosed patients seen at the oncology outpatient clinic during the 3 months we had set aside for the intervention; we received referrals for 105 patients and were able to interview 71. Only a small number, 7 of the 105 said they felt they were coping well and were not in need of a session on managing distress and learning about coping. At the final evaluation, the students were able to reach 60 patients.

Over two-thirds of the patients attended with a significant other who participated in the session by sharing both support and concerns related to family and disease issues. Seventy percent of the patients were female, and their ages ranged between 40 and 80, with an average age of 60. There was a variety of cancer types and stages.

Satisfaction and Distress Levels

The average distress level at the start of the program was 4.2. Forty-nine percent of the patients scored 5 or higher on the distress scale at the start of the project. This figure is at the high end of other screening results across Canada where the reported scores for distress levels of 5 or more range from 18 to 38 % (Carlson et al. 2004). Eight patients or 12 % scored above 7 at the program's start. At the 3-month follow-up, distress scores were significantly lower. The average distress level had dropped to 2.6. Twenty percent scored between 5 and 7 but no one scored above 7. At the evaluation, we asked if they had measured their distress since their meeting. Measuring distress using the distress thermometer is a new concept that none of the patients had been introduced to before, yet 38 % said they had continued to measure their distress using the tool.

Canadian Problem List

The number of concerns expressed ranged from 0 to 20, with a mean of 6.2. Physical problems were greater when the patient had started chemotherapy. Most patients were well prepared for chemotherapy by previously attending a class for all newly diagnosed patients that included chemo types, side effects, and delivery methods. The major physical symptoms were fatigue, pain, sleep, breathing, eating, tingling, and indigestion. The highest ranked concerns were emotional in nature: 63 % were worried, 57 % were anxious, and 53 % were afraid of the future (Refer to Table 1 for a complete list).

Eighty-two percent of the patients said they were very satisfied and recommended that the program be continued, while 18 % said they were not sure. No one

Table 1 Canadian problem list of concerns

	Ranking	Percent (%)
Worry	1	63
Nervousness	2	57
Fears	3	53
Fatigue Sadness	4	30
Pain	5	24
Sleep	6	23
Depression	7	22
Changes in appearance	8	19
Breathing	9	17
Eating Understanding my illness	10	15
Financial, insurance Tingling Dealing with children, friends	11	14
Intimacy Indigestion Knowing resources Dealing	Each 12	10

was dissatisfied with the program. Using multiple choice questions, we found that 77 % learned that coping and lowering distress were part of their care and 12 % said that they already knew that.

Only 8 % said that they did not receive useful information on handling their distress.

When we questioned them whether as a result of the session they now felt more able to cope and handle distress, only 4 % said they did not. Sixty-five percent answered yes very much and 31 % said somewhat. Most patients responded that they mostly or definitely felt a sense of control over the events in their lives, but we did not question them about this prior to the session. The booklet was found to be very useful by 65 % and somewhat by 18 %, while 17 % did not find it useful.

Thirty-six or over 50 % reported using one or more resources. About half of the resources used by the patients were ones they sought themselves, such as friends and family members. We asked three qualitative questions. One: what one thing from the meeting stood out; two, what kind of a role do you feel patients need to take in today's health-care system, and three, are there any comments you would like to add or any changes you would like to see made to the program. The qualitative questionnaire comments were positive. Comments such as the following were representative: "*greatly reduced my anxiety, enjoyed the meeting, knowing where to go for help, very helpful people to shoulder up with, answered all my questions, someone has time for me, gives you reassurance that you can do something yourself, helped by looking at my mindset, learning to be more forthright.*" The major insight for patients that emerged from the comments was the importance of being active and asking questions. Comments stressed the importance of practicing to focus on the moment and not on the distress, learning to be calm and to take care of themselves. They were pleased with how the session went and appreciated the follow-up call because they had a sense of being listened to, of being heard. Two patients suggested that the timing of the program could be earlier after diagnosis, but others commented that they felt the timing to be about right. Patients were surprised that today's health- care settings require more active participation than before, but they accepted this reality and seemed ready to take more control over their health care. For example, if test results were not forthcoming, they were prepared to call and inquire about them; if their oncologist's explanations for treatments were hard to understand, then patients would request clarification.

Discussion

It was remarkable that the mean distress level fell from 4.2 at the start of the program to 2.6 two months later. The number of patients with distress levels over 7 fell to zero from 12 %. Such improvements cannot be credited to the program alone but to a number of other contributing factors, such as patients starting chemotherapy, returning to a more familiar routine, a lessening of side effects, more time to adjust to the cancer experience, etc. Emotional problems were the most frequently cited although physical problems were also ranked as distressing to many. The nature of the problems presented by the patient and family member were highly related to current events within their social milieu, and it was the impact of having cancer on those events that concerned them. The significance of cancer within the family circle reminded us that the family is itself a unit of care with its own needs and boundaries.

We were impressed that 38 % continued to measure their distress and act on the findings, given that this was a new concept to them and that they were only introduced to it once.

We looked at time, personnel, process, content, and outcomes. The time required for the session was brief, an average of 45 min per patient plus an additional 10 min to complete a summary sheet for the oncology team. The personnel were the author and an experienced social worker. We envisage carrying out the same intervention using an operationalized format with carefully selected and trained volunteers who have themselves had a close experience with cancer. There is precedent for using volunteers in other settings for similar responsibilities (Eisner et al. 2009).

The process involved introducing the program early in the cancer trajectory before treatment started, as a part of standard care, focusing only on the patients' needs, and engaging them in recognizing their own strengths and coping strategies (Coleman and Newton 2005; Schofield et al. 2006). The content relied on active patient involvement in learning how to measure and manage their own distress, and followed the guidelines presented in the booklet. Overall, the patient-reported outcomes were highly positive. Patients were satisfied both with the program, and their subsequent ability to cope. The satisfaction felt by the patients reflects their desire to have their needs recognized. Patients felt more in control and realized their role as assertive and active members in their health care.

Recommendations

We recommend that a form of distress measurement be included in routine screening due to the relatively high levels of distress found at the start of the program. There is strong evidence that communication affects cancer patient outcomes, particularly satisfaction, psychological morbidity, and quality of life. Cancer patients rated good communication as a critical aspect of their medical care (Hack et al. 2005; Sharpley and Christie 2007). Perhaps one of the strengths of this project is the active listening by the facilitators. Facilitators did not have access to patients' charts so the patient was the only source of information. Since patients not only provided the facilitator with their most pertinent problems but worked out solutions together, the give and take of active listening took on a high level of importance. It is essential that such programs be sustainable, and able to be delivered by others than the front line oncology staff in busy, tertiary care settings. Community partnerships and resources, including volunteers, may be a realistic means to facilitate the implementation of such a program in the era of financial short falls.

Implementation and Organizational Issues

We received only 105 referrals out of a population of 630. Generally, it was the oncology nurses who decided who to refer. Most nurses explained to the patients and their families that the program was optional, thus making it easy for the patient to decline. When the oncologist recommended the program, patients willingly agreed.

There are volumes of literature that speak to the difficulty of implementing new programs into established cultures (Francke et al. 2008; Tuinman et al. 2008). How did we do with four essential requirements for successful implementation of the project? These requirements include consulting the organizational heads and front line staff, having organizational support, using a variety of strategies to ensure success, and continuous quality improvements. The chief oncologist and oncology project manager were strong advocates of the project and its potential. We did offer multifaceted targets of interventions including staff training, working with opinion leaders, policy development, audits, and ongoing feedback. We believe that our contact with the front line staff was not sufficient.

We concur with the literature that finds that programs that routinely screen and treat patients for distress are feasible, with some caveats. The introduction of the program to the front line staff is especially important in every aspect; how, when, where, how long, why, and how often (Loscalzo et al. 2011; Sollner et al. 2001). Staff were naturally reticent to fully integrate outsiders into the clinic, and in retrospect, we needed to have allocated much more time and many more resources to the introduction to the program (Andersen and Dorfman 2015). The facilitators were outsiders to the oncology clinic, and therefore were not part of the local culture. Many staff expressed the need to have resources in place that are quickly and easily accessed, and that are linked to the oncology center. This concern is reminiscent of the introduction of the pain ladder many years ago where staff were reluctant to use it, fearing they did not have the necessary resources to manage the patient's pain if it were measured.

We measured outcomes using the distress thermometer and open-ended questions, but comparisons across settings are frequently lacking. There are also many different outcomes that can be measured; we focused on patient satisfaction and levels of distress. Other outcomes of importance are the costs of running programs, the number of referrals made, long-term follow-ups, and other patient-reported outcomes. The outcomes themselves need to be assessed for their attention to quality and quantity. One general outcome that seems to be consistent among findings is that a screening process can improve communication between patients and their physicians (Fitzpatrick and Remmer 2011).

Conclusions

A brief one-session intervention cannot address all the medical, individual, sociocultural, and developmental aspects and outcomes, but it can make it easier for clinic staff to pick up on these issues and further explore them. We were pleased by the patients' responses and encouraged by their ability to learn new behaviors. With today's focus on using technology wherever possible to drive screening efforts, let us not forget that active listening to the patient's agenda, using their strengths, and helping them be active participants in their health care remain essential (Hack et al. 2005). We hope that this simple program can inspire other centers to build on it, replicate it, and assess it. Our future goal is to evaluate how well carefully selected and trained volunteers can function, using the same booklet, and following a similar protocol. Such a step is considered radical by some, yet we believe it holds the potential to expand these services to more and more patients. The volunteers would be included as members of the clinic or team, even with their limited role. A professional member of the oncology team could act as coordinator, mentor, and supervisor. These are plans for the future, and others will continue to find ways to create better person-centered care in oncology for all.

Acknowledgements The author would like to gratefully acknowledge her colleague, Sandra Hardy, MSW who partnered with her in the development and implementation of the program.

References

Andersen, B. L., & Dorfman, C. S. (2015). Evidence-based psychosocial treatment in the community: Considerations for dissemination and implementation. *Psycho-Oncology*, n/a–n/a. doi:10.1002/pon.3864

Andersen, B. L., Yang, H. C., Farrar, W. B., Golden-Kreutz, D. M., Emery, C. F., Thornton, L. M., & Carson, W. E, 3rd. (2008). Psychologic intervention improves survival for breast cancer patients: A randomized clinical trial. *Cancer, 113*(12), 3450–3458. doi:10.1002/cncr.23969

Bruera, E., Kuehn, N., Miller, M. J., Selmser, P., & Macmillan, K. (1991). The Edmonton symptom assessment system (ESAS): A simple method for the assessment of palliative care patients. *Journal of Palliative Care, 7*(2), 6–9.

Bultz, B. D., & Johansen, C. (2011). Screening for distress, the 6th vital sign: Where are we, and where are we going? *Psychooncology, 20*(6), 569–571. doi:10.1002/pon.1986

Carlson, L. E., Angen, M., Cullum, J., Goodey, E., Koopmans, J., Lamont, L., & Bultz, B. D. (2004). High levels of untreated distress and fatigue in cancer patients. *British Journal of Cancer, 90*(12), 2297–2304. doi:10.1038/sj.bjc.6601887

Coleman, M. T., & Newton, K. S. (2005). Supporting self-management in patients with chronic illness. *American Family Physician, 72*(8), 1503–1510.

Edgar, L. (2010). *Mastering the art of coping in good times and bad*. Canada: Copelindaedgar.

Eisner, D., Grimm, R. T., Maynard, S., & Washburn, S. (2009). The new volunteer workforce. *Stanford Social Innovation Review*.

Fitch, M. I. (2009). Supportive care framework: Theoretical underpinnings. *Supportive Care Framework: A Foundation for Person-Centered Care* (Pappin Communications).

Fitzpatrick, T. R., & Remmer, J. (2011). Needs, expectations and attendance among participants of a cancer wellness centre in Montreal, Quebec. *Journal of Cancer Survivorship, 5*(3), 235–246. doi:10.1007/s11764-011-0176-8

Francke, A., Smit, M., de Veer, A., & Mistiaen, P. (2008). Factors influencing the implementation of clinical guidelines for health care professionals: A systematic meta-review. *BMC Medical Informatics and Decision Making, 8*(1), 1–11. doi:10.1186/1472-6947-8-38

Giesler, R. B., Given, B., Given, C. W., Rawl, S., Monahan, P., Burns, D., & Champion, V. (2005). Improving the quality of life of patients with prostate carcinoma: a randomized trial testing the efficacy of a nurse-driven intervention. *Cancer, 104*(4), 752–762. doi:10.1002/cncr.21231

Grant, M., Economou, D., Ferrell, B., & Uman, G. (2012). Educating health care professionals to provide institutional changes in cancer survivorship care. *Journal of Cancer Education, 27*(2), 226–232. doi:10.1007/s13187-012-0314-7

Hack, T. F., Degner, L. F., & Parker, P. A. (2005). The communication goals and needs of cancer patients: a review. *Psychooncology, 14*(10), 831–845; discussion 846–837. doi:10.1002/pon.949

Hewitt, M., Herdman, R., & Holland, J. (2004). The effectiveness of psychosocial interventions for women with breast cancer. In M. Hewitt, R. Herdman & J. Holland (Eds.), *Meeting psychosocial needs of women with breast cancer* (pp. 95–132). USA: The National Academies Press. Retrieved from http://www.ncbi.nlm.nih.gov/books/NBK215944/

Jacobsen, P. B. (2009). Promoting evidence-based psychosocial care for cancer patients. *Psychooncology, 18*(1), 6–13. doi:10.1002/pon.1468

Jacobsen, P. B., Shibata, D., Siegel, E. M., Lee, J. H., Fulp, W. J., Alemany, C., & Malafa, M. (2011). Evaluating the quality of psychosocial care in outpatient medical oncology settings using performance indicators. *Psychooncology, 20*(11), 1221–1227. doi:10.1002/pon.1849

Lauver, D. R., Connolly-Nelson, K., & Vang, P. (2007). Stressors and coping strategies among female cancer survivors after treatments. *Cancer Nursing, 30*(2), 101–111. doi:10.1097/01.NCC.0000265003.56817.2c

Lazarus, R. S., & Folkman, S. (1984). *Stress, appraisal, and coping*: Springer Publishing Company.

Loscalzo, M., Clark, K. L., & Holland, J. (2011). Successful strategies for implementing biopsychosocial screening. *Psychooncology, 20*(5), 455–462. doi:10.1002/pon.1930

Meyer, T., & Mark, M. (1995). Effects of psychosocial interventions with adult cancer patients; a meta-analysis of randomized experiments. *Health Psychology, 14*(2), 101–108.

Miaskowski, C. (2004). Gender differences in pain, fatigue, and depression in patients with cancer. *Journal of National Cancer Institute Monographs, 32*, 139–143. doi:10.1093/jncimonographs/lgh024

Schofield, P., Carey, M., Bonevski, B., & Sanson-Fisher, R. (2006). Barriers to the provision of evidence-based psychosocial care in oncology. *Psychooncology, 15*(10), 863–872. doi:10.1002/pon.1017

Sharpley, C. F., & Christie, D. R. H. (2007). 'How I was then and how I am now': Current and retrospective self-reports of anxiety and depression in Australian women with breast cancer. *Psycho-Oncology, 16*(8), 752–762. doi:10.1002/pon.1125

Silver, J. K., & Baima, J. (2013). Cancer prehabilitation: An opportunity to decrease treatment-related morbidity, increase cancer treatment options, and improve physical and psychological health outcomes. *American Journal of Physical Medicine Rehabilitation, 92*(8), 715–727. doi:10.1097/PHM.0b013e31829b4afe

Sollner, W., DeVries, A., Steixner, E., Lukas, P., Sprinzl, G., Rumpold, G., & Maislinger, S. (2001). How successful are oncologists in identifying patient distress, perceived social support, and need for psychosocial counselling? *British Journal of Cancer, 84*(2), 179–185. doi:10.1054/bjoc.2000.1545

Spiegel, D., Butler, L. D., Giese-Davis, J., Koopman, C., Miller, E., DiMiceli, S., & Kraemer, H. C. (2007). Effects of supportive-expressive group therapy on survival of patients with metastatic breast cancer: A randomized prospective trial. *Cancer, 110*(5), 1130–1138. doi:10.1002/cncr.22890

Stanton, A. L. (2012). What happens now? Psychosocial care for cancer survivors after medical treatment completion. *Journal of Clinical Oncology, 30*(11), 1215–1220. doi:10.1200/jco.2011.39.7406

Sundar, V., Fox, S. W., & Phillips, K. G. (2013). Transitions in caregiving: Evaluating a person-centered approach to supporting family caregivers in the community. *Journal of Gerontological Social Work, 57*(6–7), 750–765. doi:10.1080/01634372.2013.847885

Tuinman, M. A., Gazendam-Donofrio, S. M., & Hoekstra-Weebers, J. E. (2008). Screening and referral for psychosocial distress in oncologic practice: Use of the Distress Thermometer. *Cancer, 113*(4), 870–878. doi:10.1002/cncr.23622

Vos, J., Craig, M., & Cooper, M. (2015). Existential therapies: A meta-analysis of their effects on psychological outcomes. *Journal of Consulting Clinical Psychology, 83*(1), 115–128. doi:10.1037/a0037167

Whitney, R. L., Bell, J. F., Bold, R. J., & Joseph, J. G. (2015). Mental health needs and service use in a national sample of adult cancer survivors in the USA: Has psychosocial care improved? *Psychooncology, 24*(1), 80–88. doi:10.1002/pon.3569

Chapter 3
Latino Cancer Survivors: The Old and the Young

Tanya R. Fitzpatrick

Introduction

Latino survivors of cancer, especially the elderly and young children, have suffered from numerous barriers to treatment as a result of economic oppression, physical health, and psychological problems. This chapter explores quality of life issues among children, adolescents and older Latinos and how culturally appropriate interventions attempt to address the physical, social and psychological barriers faced by this underserved population. Long after successful treatment, survivors are often faced with the physical and mental toll of their diagnosis (Ceballos et al. 2015). For example, factors such as poverty, language barriers, lack of proper health insurance and screening for cancer create a greater risk for the advanced stages of the disease once diagnosed (Farone et al. 2008). Physical health-related symptoms of cancer affecting quality of life outcomes are pain, fatigue and physical limitations brought on by the short and long-term effects of chemotherapy, radiation and surgery (Fitzpatrick and Farone 2011). It is not surprising that the survival rate for Latinos is lower than for non-Hispanic whites as they wait longer for treatment even after diagnosis due in part to limited information and access (Wu et al. 2001). However, research has shown that targeted interventions have a beneficial effect on psychological and physical health among Latino cancer survivors (Ceballos et al. 2015).

Although some previous studies have addressed social support and physical activity interventions, they have mainly focused on Latina breast cancer survivors (Ashing-Giwa et al. 2006; Sheppard et al. 2008; Welsh et al. 2005). This chapter is unique because few studies have examined the relationship between various therapeutic interventions as they relate to the quality of life among different age

T.R. Fitzpatrick (✉)
Professor Emeritus, Department of Social Work, Arizona State University,
449 Mount Pleasant Ave, Westmount, QC H3Y3G9, Canada
e-mail: tanya.fitzpatrick@asu.edu

T.R. Fitzpatrick (ed.), *Treating Vulnerable Populations of Cancer Survivors: A Biopsychosocial Approach*, DOI 10.1007/978-3-319-32364-0_3

groups of Latino cancer survivors experiencing different types of cancer (Fitzpatrick and Farone 2011). Quality of life (QOL) can be defined as the individual's subjective evaluations of physical and psychological health and also by their appraisal and satisfaction with their present level of functioning. The ultimate goal is to shed further light and understanding by exploring existing theoretical perspectives and literature describing interventions such as physical activities, leisure and household activities, church-related activities, social support groups and educational programs. The aims of the chapter will be addressed by focusing on the following:

1. Demographic information
2. Theoretical perspectives specific to Latinos with cancer
3. Review of the literature on various therapeutic interventions
4. Implications for clinical practice and future research.

Basic Demographic Information

The terms "Hispanic" and "Latino/a" are used to refer to persons of Hispanic origin. Much of the research on cancer statistics has been directed towards Latinos in the U.S. and very little research has specifically focused on Latino survivors living in Canada. However, more recent investigations do include both Canada and the U.S. (Canadian Cancer Statistics Publication 2015; Singh and Miller 2004). According to the American Cancer Society (2012–2014), 50.5 million Americans (16 % of the U.S. population) are identified as Hispanics or Latino. By the year 2050, elderly Hispanics/Latinos will total 12 million, eleven times as many as in 2009 (Intercultural Cancer Council 2011; US Census Bureau 2011). As described by Wu et al. (2001), in Fitzpatrick and Farone (2011), the cancer survival rate is lower for Hispanics than for non-Hispanic whites and elderly Hispanics have less information about screening, health prevention and insurance and are diagnosed at later stages of the disease.

Many of the studies focusing on Latinos with cancer have been directed to women with breast cancer (Budhrani et al. 2014; Yanez et al. 2011; Shephard et al. 2007). Yet, older Hispanics are less likely to be screened for breast and cervical cancer than their younger counterparts. Latina women aged 50 and older have the lowest mammogram utilization rates and women 18 and older have the lowest Pap test utilization than other racial and ethnic groups (Intercultural Cancer Council 2011). In addition, elderly Hispanics have a greater number of functional disabilities than elderly non-Hispanics, especially from cancer-related outcomes. This points out the need for continuing education directed toward oncology professionals to enable them to practice more efficiently by addressing the specific challenges of this population.

Cancer in Latino Children and Adolescence

Cancer in children is rare but in 2014, it is estimated that 15,780 have been diagnosed. Although the survival rate has increased for all types of cancer, nearly 2000 children die of cancer each year in the U.S. thus indicating the need for effective treatments to further reduce mortality (Ward et al. 2014). However, Latino and other minority groups of adolescents and young adults have not received the same survival rates as in older adults and younger children. Of the 724 AYAs studied, 36 % were Hispanics and although, being a male, increasing age, and advanced cancer were associated with elevated mortality, the survival disparity for race/ethnicity existed despite equal access to care.

Few studies are available on statistics among young children and adolescents of Hispanic origin with cancer published in either the U.S. or Canada. However, one study that was published in São Paulo, Brazil (2010), including 10 children and 8 adolescents between the ages of 8 and 18 years, sought to understand the physical and psychological effects of chemotherapy from the perspective of children and adolescents (Chico de Cicogna et al. 2010). Results indicated that chemotherapy is the most employed treatment. The responses from the children interviewed remembered the experience as that of suffering and pain but over time as recovery and cure mainly as a result of the chemotherapy. Quality of life stands out as a priority for the families and their children who have cancer. Several major themes related to quality of life were discussed such as loneliness, isolation, loss of normal childhood, decreased employment opportunities among adolescents, physical discomfort, disability, and emotional responses (Chico de Cicogna et al. 2010).

Theoretical Perspectives

Many of the theories on ethnic and cultural perspectives that were mentioned earlier may also apply to the elderly, young children, and adolescent Latino cancer survivors. Although, not specific to Latinos, there are several that relate to older adults from minority populations. They are presented in more detail here to further clarify and highlight the experience of cancer and quality of life among these groups. The *double jeopardy hypothesis* (Butler et al. 1991; Dowd and Bengston 1978) was developed to accommodate differences and disparities between Blacks and Whites (Butler et al. 1991), yet it is applicable to other minority groups. This hypothesis is characterized as a double burden resulting from "devaluation in status in society" (Alemán et al. 2000, p. 6). A triple jeopardy scenario can also be applied to those being elderly, being female, and being from a minority group plus having low economic status. *Modernization theory* postulates that as each ethnic society modernizes and becomes more industrialized, the less status the elders' position in the family carries (Cowgill and Holmes 1972; Markides and Mindel 1987), This may be true in America today as Latinos are becoming a large part of society and changes in the traditional family structure are evident. For example, some elders are now being placed in long-term care facilities when younger family members feel that they can no longer take care of them at home similar to their American and Canadian counterparts. *Assimilation theory* (Markides and Mindel 1987) is also explained by Alemán et al. (2000) in that ethnic and minority status becomes temporary, as when one moves up the socioeconomic ladder towards a middle-class position, cultural distinctiveness becomes absent. This is contrary to the process of *acculturation* and *cultural pluralism* (Healey 1996; Fitzpatrick 2000; Tran et al. 1996) as now many ethnic groups similar to the Hispanics who have been in America for generations continue to follow their traditions and customs as well as those of the mainstream. *Acculturation* is a process based on language and education (Tran et al. 1996), which for many elderly Latinos can be a major issue and barrier for seeking appropriate health screening and treatment for cancer.

Alemán (2000) in Alemán et al. (2000) explains the system of "*compadrazco*" as a trait in which Mexican American families continue to rely heavily on extended support that is intergenerational, which can include non-blood relatives. The family usually assists in the elder's health care decisions that value the group over the individual. This in most cases can be beneficial for the elder; however, service providers must understand this important family dynamic in order for assistance to be helpful for the family. "*Personalisma*" is another important trait common to most Latinos (Alemán 2000). It is customary and important for the elder to feel that the provider is a trusting person and one who is willing to share his or her person information. If this is not the case, the elder may not return for much needed assistance. For example, the elder may ask the health-care professional personal questions such as, "How old are you? Do you speak Spanish?" or "How many children do you have?" This may seem too personal for the professional but it is essential to "self-disclose" to a certain extent to foster a good working and trusting relationship between the provider and the elder client. While these perspectives are not exhaustive, they do provide further understanding as to how necessary it is for healthcare providers to assess cultural values and make appropriate interventions to older and younger Hispanics and their family members (Alemán 2000).

The Cancer Experience Among Latino Children and Adolescents

Most of the literature on the experience of cancer among children and adolescents addressing conceptual perspectives is directed toward the general population (Bruce 2006; Haase 2004; Simon et al. 2003; Stuber et al. 1997). Few researchers have focused on Latino children and adolescents with the exception of a group of researchers from São Paulo, Brazil. In a study examining motherhood among Hispanic children with cancer, Moreira and Angelo (2008) introduce the perspective of *Symbolic Interactionism.* The main ideas are based on the process of interaction among individuals in which meaning is found between human beings. Therefore, the meaning of the cancer experience for mothers of children is found with interactions between the mother, the disease, the child or adolescents, and the health care team. This interaction includes *interpretation* of important life experiences, which will enable further knowledge and understanding of the reality of the situation (Moreira and Angelo 2008). This will bring a new direction to the lives of the mothers who are caring for a child with an often fatal disease. Another study by Chico de Cicogna et al. (2010) focusing on the experience of chemotherapy and quality of life found revealed several major themes such as loneliness and isolation, loss of normal childhood, decreased enjoyment of food, physical discomfort and disability and emotional responses to cancer. These themes are useful for oncology professionals to understand the experience of the disease in order to help Latino children and adolescents with cancer "to find new ways of coping and living well." (p. 2).

Finally, the development of interdisciplinary healthcare to Latino children and adolescents with cancer in pain situations is examined from the perspective of the *Complexity Paradigm.* This paradigm attempts to address the multidimensional characteristics and the complexity of the reality of the experience without isolating the biological, psychological and social dimensions (Menossi et al. 2008). For example, the pain associated with cancer is seen as a complex phenomenon for healthcare professionals who are attempting to understand the work involved in the process of providing healthcare, and to transform the knowledge into collective actions for children and their families of Hispanic origin.

Age and Culturally Appropriate Interventions

Interventions designed to improve health and quality of life for vulnerable populations of Latino cancer survivors will be explored along with implications for appropriate clinical practice and future research.

Physical Activities: Regular physical activity is said to enhance health and physical functioning in older populations (Satariano et al. 2002). Specific to cancer survivors, different types of sports and physical activities were related to activity levels before and after a diagnosis of breast cancer. For example, decreased activity levels were associated with poorer quality of life after the diagnosis. The need to increase physical activity may provide physical benefits to women with a higher perceived risk of breast cancer (Audrain et al. 2001). A recent study by Fitzpatrick and Farone (2011) indicated that leisure activity participation and especially, household activities were significantly related to self-reported health, cutting down on activities, and depressive symptoms among older Mexican Americans with cancer living in the southwest USA. Household activities such as cleaning the house, preparing meals (light household activities), carrying water and wood, repairs, caring for others, and gardening (heavy household activities), were valued as important activities among Mexican elders.

Although not focusing on Latino elderly, Fitzpatrick et al. (2012) found that physical fitness activities such as any body movement produced by skeletal muscles that results in energy expenditure on a daily basis, is said to help reduce the cognitive effects of chemotherapy among older cancer survivors over the short and long term. Another study promoting the beneficial affects of physical activities by Leimanis and Fitzpatrick (2014) revealed that physical activities preformed at a cancer support center and others preformed at home had a significant effect on distress, in that distress was reduced among the group of cancer survivors.

Support Groups

The *family systems and sociocultural framework* that integrates culture and social class relates to family-focused interventions for families facing cancer (Marshall et al. 2011). Family-focused interventions emphasizing social class (SES), especially among low income families, are necessary for health care professionals to understand in order to provide guidance to cancer survivors and their families. For example, intervention approaches would include the following suggestions; (1) *Flexibility* is needed when working with culturally diverse and low income populations in regards to scheduling of interventions such as health appointments, school, work, and other family responsibilities, (2) Interventions should consider *language* differences and the need to provide bilingual interpreters and providers, (3) *Travel and transportation* may be costly for low income and immigrant families, therefore bringing information into schools and community health centers may be more convenient and assessable, (4) As *financial concerns* may be present, information regarding financial resources should be made available as part of a cancer education program, (5) To create a *child and family-friendly environment*, allowing time for eating and food preparation should be included in the overall program interventions, and finally, (6) *Follow-up and referrals* to community agencies is needed. "Perhaps scheduling a Saturday morning using in-home cancer education programs may result in a referral to a family support groups or even a hospice program for example" (Marshall et al. 2011, p. 91).

In line with the recommendations presented from Marshall et al. (2011), Munet-Vilaró (2004) discusses the delivery of culturally competent interventions for Latino children with cancer and their families. There is a scarcity of research that investigates the factors that can influence the responses to cancer. It is suggested that in order to practice culturally competent care, clinicians (eg., nurses, social workers, oncologists) collaboration between multidisciplinary teams should provide increased awareness and knowledge to help serve the needs of this population. Besides language and information dissemination, clinicians should acquaint themselves with a comprehensive understanding of issues of childhood cancer such as the etiology of specific types of cancer, different treatments, and community resources, and how this knowledge may reflect differences in cultural values and outcomes among Latino children and their families. For example, understanding cultural values such as fatalism, death and dying, suffering, along with differences in coping strategies, can lead to culturally competent interventions that address more adequately the needs of this underserved population (Munet-Vilaró 2004).

Senior Centers

Although not directly related to younger age groups with cancer, participation in senior centers has been shown to moderate stress-related distress among Latino elders (Farone et al. 2005). The results of these studies revealed that for those Latinos who were experiencing stressful life situations, participation in senior center activities lowered their psychological distress. Community Senior Centers provide an array of social supports for older adults and have been "conceptualized as a resource that provides a variety of services, including health, social, nutrition and meal plans, education, and recreational activities, which provide ample opportunities for social interaction" (Farone et al. 2005, p. 66). These centers also serve immigrant populations with cancer. Senior Centers can be seen as an intervention strategy to moderate the harmful impact of stressful life situations (Fitzpatrick et al. 2005a, b). Therefore, the promotion of Senior Centers by professionals can serve as a useful community support for Latino elders with cancer and their families (Farone et al. 2005). Regardless, linguistic and cultural barriers make the use and access to community supports such as senior centers a greater challenge for Latino cancer survivors.

Focus Groups

Ceballos et al. (2015) conducted bilingual and bicultural focus groups by "*promotores*" and face-to-face interviews to address a wide range of burdens that Mexican American cancer survivors and their families experience such as depression, isolation, fear of recurrence, stress and changes in body image. This intervention strategy proved to be beneficial to the cancer survivors who participated. The support groups provided an opportunity for healing and the ability to better understand and cope with their disease on a daily basis. A key role in the successful intervention was played by the promotores, which should be taken into account by oncology professionals when providing future supportive interventions for this group of cancer survivors (Ceballos et al. 2015).

Educational and Church-Based Interventions

Between 1998 and 2001, two church-based interventions aimed at reducing the cancer screening rates were introduced to Latinas with breast cancer living in Colorado, U.S. The objectives of The Tepeyac Project attempted to compare two Tepeyac interventions on the mammogram rates of Latinas and non-Latina whites in the Medicaid fee-for-service program (Welsh et al. 2005). There were 209 churches included in the study that provided educational printed material in Spanish and English. The second intervention involved peer counselors (*The Promotora Intervention*) in which the subjects received personalized education. The effects of the interventions on the rates of mammogram use were assessed between the two groups aged 50–64 years already enrolled in the Medicaid program. The results revealed that the personalized community-based education (*Promotora Intervention*) was effective but only modestly for increasing breast cancer screening rates among the two Latina groups. The authors point out that other services and supports along with church-based education may be necessary (Welsh et al. 2005).

The *Nueva Luz* is an educational intervention developed to address quality of life among Latina breast cancer survivors in the City of Hope, Duarte, CA. The main goal of the program was to provide strategies to assist in the transition to survivorship (Jaurez et al. 2014). The English and Spanish educational intervention was used to access psychosocial issues, which utilized a purposive sample of eight Latina breast cancer survivors. The results indicate that the one-on-one approach, which provides bilingual printed information plus verbal instruction from a bilingual and culturally competent professional, can serve as an effective resource in helping Latina women with breast cancer transition into survivorship and improve quality of life.

Finally, using art therapy as a psychosocial intervention, six young women with a recent diagnosis of breast cancer explored the multi-faceted artist's fold book in an art therapy group at a community cancer support center in Montreal (Laux 2015). The results revealed that young women with breast cancer benefited from participation in weekly art groups allowing themselves to reveal their feelings and concerns in a safe and supportive environment thus helping to improve their quality of life. This would suggest that an innovative intervention such as art therapy would also serve as an effective means for self-awareness among young children and adolescent cancer survivors.

Summary and Discussion

This chapter has highlighted some of the important survivorship issues, which present considerable challenges for Latinos with cancer, especially among the young and older age groups. Demographic information, theoretical perspectives, and innovative therapeutic interventions have been presented in an attempt to shed light on the cultural context in the delivery of appropriate educational programs and services. Despite improvements in survival rates and more advanced treatments, the cancer survival rate remains lower for Hispanics than for non-Hispanic whites. Elderly Hispanics have less information about screening, health prevention and insurance and are diagnosed at later stages of the disease (Fitzpatrick and Farone 2011; Wu et al. 2001). As described earlier in the chapter, many of the studies focusing on Latinos with cancer have been directed to the delivery of psychosocial services and programs for women with breast cancer (Budhrani et al. 2014; Yanez et al. 2011; Shephard et al. 2007). Yet these educational and supportive interventions are just as relevant for all ages of Latinos despite the fact the older Hispanics as a group experience greater challenges and have less access to education, health and screening services and face limitations due to language barriers and functional disabilities. Young children and adolescents from Latino backgrounds are just as likely as their older counterparts to experience the same barriers and difficulties during survivorship. Furthermore, adolescents and young adults from all racial and ethnic backgrounds (AYAs) continue to experience inferior survival rates compared to older adults and younger children.

Leukemia is the most common cancer in all children. Hispanic children have the highest rate of leukemia of any ethnic group, even higher than African American children (American Cancer Society 2012–2014). The survival rate has improved among Hispanic children, however, it remains lower compared to non-Hispanic children for all types of leukemia. It is suggested that access to treatment may account for some of the differences, yet these differences are also apparent in clinical trials with those who have equal treatment. The disparity may also be "due to high-risk leukemia types among Hispanic children" (American Cancer Society 2012–2014, p. 13). Symptoms affecting quality of life among all cancer survivors and especially in Latino adolescents and children include post traumatic stress syndrome (PSTD) (Bruce 2006; Stuber et al. 1997), pain, dyspnea, nose bleeds, seizures and fatigue (Van Cleve et al. 2012; Menossi et al. 2008), fear, anxiety and depression (Stuber et al. 1997).

The cancer screening rates for all Americans are relatively low; however, people from racial and ethnic minorities have the lowest rates together with those with low income, the elderly and the medically underserved (Centers for Disease Control and Prevention 2001). Many older adults with cancer tend to be underserved and the majority are women from different ethnic groups. Appropriate palliation is less frequent and they receive less aggressive therapy. Current methods of care are often based on assumptions and stereotypical thinking (Surbone et al. 2007).

Implications for Clinical Practice and Future Research

The development of culturally competent care for Latino children with cancer and their families should be first and foremost in importance for oncology and health care providers (Munet-Vilaró 2004). It is important for clinicians to respond appropriately to the specific needs and behaviors that are unique to their cultural norms. For many Latino families facing a life-threatening disease, *Fatalismo* is a way of coping, which many Latinos experience as a deep acceptance of the disease and is therefore beyond their control (Farone et al. 2008). It is suggested that clinicians communicate to family members with translators when necessary, and that despite their resignation and beliefs, it is expected that the best oncology care from professionals will be provided to their child. Many child and family visits take place in the home following lengthy hospital stays, yet it can be threatening when health care providers, seen as strangers, enter the home. Parents of children and their elderly family members may not speak English, however if a translator is available it can eliminate fears of mistrust (Alemán 2000). Alemán states that the concept of trust and mutual respect between the healthcare provider and the family is of utmost importance, especially when working with children, adolescents, and elderly family members with cancer, however, this may take considerable patience and time from the healthcare provider. All members of the family need to be involved, and in most cases they insist, however, they remain in need of on-going communication, education and understanding during the survivorship experience. Although Latino adolescents have been learning English in schools and have become acculturated sooner than their elder family members, they still require information regarding their disease and an opportunity to express their concerns and fears and to also have the opportunity to be involved in decisions regarding their treatment plan.

The need to remain in control and assist in making decisions about treatment is therefore an important aspect when working with adolescents. The Adolescent Resilience Model (Haase 2004) is an example of interventions that address positive health strategies such as hope and coping together with positive support from family, friends and the healthcare team. Considering the challenges in understanding the complexity of working with Latino children, adolescents, the elderly and family members, especially when fate, suffering, resignation and differences in coping styles exist is essential for providers (Munet-Vilaró 2004). Establishing effective interdisciplinary communication is necessary to address the multiple dimensions that compose the healthcare for underserved groups of Latinos during the entire survivorship process.

Future research and policy interventions should focus on enhancing community supports by attempting to include bilingual and bicultural staff and clinicians and targeting appropriate health services, social supports and acculturation needs. Young children and adolescents should be directed toward peer support activities and services that address academic and job-related issues, along with health and disease education for their families. Future research should continue to address issues of isolation, loneliness, and other psychological needs of elderly Latinos with cancer including education and language acquisition plus ways to facilitate the survivorship needs. This will contribute to a more optimistic sense of well-being and quality of life thus reflecting on the individuals ability to remain independent and continue to live in the community for as long as possible (Fitzpatrick 2000). Additionally, and of equal importance, future investigations are needed to evaluate the education and training of oncology and healthcare professionals focusing not only on the disease and medical treatment but on the psychosocial needs. This will provide more culturally competent care for Latino cancer survivors. Oncology practitioners and healthcare workers should remain open to new knowledge, differing beliefs and innovative ways to face the numerous challenges that cancer survivors endure, which will do well to ensure the health and well-being of those we serve (Damskey 2000).

References

Alemán, S. (2000). Mexican American elders. In S. Alemán, T. R. Fitzpatrick, T. V. Tran, & E. Gonzalus (Eds.), *Therapeutic interventions with ethnic elders: Health and social issues* (pp. 139–148). New York, London: The Hayworth Press.

Alemán, S., Fitzpatrick, T. R., Tran, T. V., & Gonzalus, E. (Eds.). (2000). *Therapeutic interventions with ethnic elders: Health and social issues*. New York, London: The Hayworth Press.

American Cancer Society. (2012–2014). Cancer facts and figures for Hispanic Latinos. Atlanta, GA: American Cancer Society.

Ashing-Giwa, K. T., Padilla, G. V., Bohorquez, D. E., Tejero, S. J., & Garcia, M. (2006). Understanding the breast cancer expectations of Latina women. *Journal of Psychosocial Oncol, 24*(3), 19–52.

Audrain, J., Schwartz, M., Herrera, J., Goldman, P., & Bush, A. (2001). Physical activity in first-degree relatives of breast cancer. *Journal of Behavioral Medicine, 24*, 587–603.

Bruce, M. (2006). A systematic and conceptual review of posttraumatic stress in childhood cancer survivors and their parents. *Clinical Psychology Review, 26*, 233–256.

Budhrani, P. H., Lengacher, C. A., Kip, K. E., Tofthagen, C., & Jim, H. (2014). Minority breast cancer survivors: The association between Race/ethnicity, objective sleep disturbances, and physical and psychological symptoms. *Nursing Research and Practice*, 11. http://dx.doi.org/10.1155/2014/858403

Butler, R. N., Lewis, M., & Sunderland, T. (1991). *Aging and mental health: Positive psychosocial and biomedical approaches*. New York: Macmillan Publishing Company.

Canadian Cancer Statistics Publication. (2015). In Canadian Cancer Society, 2015. Info@cis.cancer.ca.

Ceballos, R. M., Molina, Y., Ibarra, G., Escareno, M., & Marchello, N. (2015). Design, development, and feasibility of a Spanish-language cancer support group. *Support Care Cancer*. doi:10.1007/s00520-014-2549-9

Centers for Disease Control and Prevention. (2001). National breast and cervical cancer early detection program (NBCCEDP). *Cancer Screening-United States, 2010*. MMWR2012 *61*(3), 41–45.

Chico de Cicogna, E., Nasciment, L. C., & Garcia, R. A. (2010). Children and adolescents with cancer. *Revista latino-americana de enfermagem, 18*(5) (September/October 2010). http://dx.dol.org/10.1590/SO104-11692010000500005

Cowgill, D. O., & Holmes, L. (1972). *Aging and modernization*. New York: Appleton-Century-Crofts.

Damskey, M. (2000). Views and visions: Moving toward culturally competent practice. In S. Alemán, T. R. Fitzpatrick, T. V. Tran, & E. Gonzalus (Eds.), *Therapeutic interventions with ethnic elders: Health and social issues* (pp. 195–208). New York, London: The Hayworth Press.

Dowd, J. J., & Bengston, V. (1978). Aging in minority populations: An examination of the double jeopardy hypothesis. *Journal of Gerontology, 33*, 427–436.

Farone, D. W., Fitzpatrick, T. R., & Bushfield, S. Y. (2008). Hope, locus of control, and quality of health among elder Latina cancer survivors. *Social Work in Health Care, 46*, 51–70.

Farone, D. W., Fitzpatrick, T. R., & Tran, T. V. (2005). Use of Senior Centers as a stress-coping strategy among Latino elders. *The Journal of Gerontological Social Work, 46*, 65–83.

Fitzpatrick, T. R. (2000). Elderly Russian Jewish immigrants. In S. Alemán, T. R. Fitzpatrick, T. V. Tran, & E. Gonzalus (Eds.), *Therapeutic interventions with ethnic elders: Health and social issues*. New York, London: The Hayworth Press.

Fitzpatrick, T. R., Edgar, L., & Holcroft, C. (2012). Assessing the relationship between physical fitness activities, cognitive health and quality of life among older breast cancer survivors. *Journal of Psychosocial Oncology, 30*, 556–572.

Fitzpatrick, T. R., & Farone, D. W. (2011). Leisure, household activities and health among Mexican American elders with cancer. *Journal of Psychosocial Oncology, 29*, 199–214.

Fitzpatrick, T. R., Gitelson, K., Andereck, K., & Mesbur, E. S. (2005a). Social support and health among a Senior Center population in Southern, Ontario, Canada. *Social Work and Health Care, 40*, 15–37.

Fitzpatrick, T. R., McCabe, J., Gitelson, R., & Andereck, K. (2005b). Factors effecting perceived social and health benefits among senior center participants. *Activities, Adaptation and Aging, 30*, 23–45.

Haase, J. E. (2004). The adolescent resilience model as a guide to interventions. *Journal of Pediatric Nursing, 21*, 289–299.

Healey, J. F. (1996). *Race, ethnicity and gender in the U.S.* Thousand Oaks, CA: Pine Forge Press.

Intercultural Cancer Council. (2011). Native Hawaiians/Pacific Islanders Cancer. In *Cancer facts sheet*. http://ICCNetwork.org

Jaurez, G., Mayorga, L., Hurria, A., & Ferrell, B. (2014). Survivorship education for Latina breast cancer survivors: Empowering survivors through education. *Psicooncologia, 10*, 57–66. doi:10.5209/rev%20PSIC.2013.v10.41947

Laux, K. (2015). Exploring the artist's book: How art therapy can benefit the quality of life of young adult breast cancer survivors (in preparation).

Leimanis, M. L., & Fitzpatrick, T. R. (2014). Physical activities and distress among participants of a cancer wellness centre: A community-based pilot study. *International Journal of Physical Medicine & Rehabilitation, 2*(3), 1–8.

Markides, K. S., & Mindel, C. H. (1987). *Aging and ethnicity*. Newbury Park, CA: Sage Publications.

Marshall, C. A., Larkey, L. K., Curran, M. A., Weihs, K. L., Bager, T. A., Armin, J., & Garcia, F. (2011). Considerations of culture and social class for families facing cancer: The need for a new model for health promotion and psychosocial intervention. *Family Systems Health, 29*, 81–94.

Menossi, M. J., Garcia de Lima, R. A., & Corréa, A. K. (2008). Pain and the challenge of interdisciplinarity in child care. *Revista latino-americana de enfermagem, 1, 6*(3) (May-June 2008). http://dx.dol.org/10.1590/SO104-11692008000300025

Moreira, P. L., Angelo, M. (2008). Becoming a mother of a child with cancer: Building motherhood. *Revista latino-americana de enfermagem, 16*(3) (May-June 2008). http://dx.dol.org/10.1590/SO104-11692008000300004

Munet-Vilaró, F. (2004). Delivery of culturally competent care to children with cancer and their families—The Latino Experience. *Journal of Pediatric Oncology Nursing, 21*, 155–159.

Satariano, W. A., Haight, T. J., & Tager, I. B. (2002). Living arrangements and participation in leisure-time activities in an older population. *Journal of Aging and Health, 14*, 427–451.

Shephard, F. A., Crawley, J., Van Houtte, P., Postmus, P. E., Carney, D., Chansky, K., Shaikh, Z., & Goldstraw, P. (2007). The international association for the study of lung cancer staging project: Proposals regarding the clinical staging of small cell lung cancer in the forthcoming 7th Ed. of the tumor, node, metastasis classification for lung cancer. *Journal of Thoracic Cancer, 2*, 1067–1077. doi:10.1097/JTO.06013e31815bdcOd

Sheppard, V. B. Figueiredo, M., Canar, J., Goodman, M., Caicedo, L., Kaufman, A., et al. (2008). Latina a Latina: Developing a breast cancer decision support intervention. *Psycho-Oncology, 17,* 383–391. doi:10.1002/pon.1239

Simon, C., Zyzanski, S., Eder, M., Raiz, P., Kodish, E. D., & Siminoff, L. A. (2003). Groups potentially at risk for making poorly informed decisions about entry into clinical trials for childhood cancer. *Journal of Clinical Psychology, 21,* 2173–2178. doi:10.1200/JCO.2003.03.003

Singh, G. K., & Miller, B. A. (2004). Health, life expectancy, and mortality patterns among immigrant populations in the U.S. *Canadian Journal of Public Health, 95*(3), 1–24.

Stuber, M. L., Kazek, A. E., Meeske, K., Baraket, L., Guthrie, D., Garnier, H., et al. (1997). Predictors of post-traumatic stress symptoms in childhood cancer survivors. *Pediatrics, 100,* 958–964.

Surbone, A., Kagawa-Singer, M., Terret, C., & Baider, L. (2007). The illness trajectory of elderly cancer patients across cultures: SIOG position paper. *Annuals of Oncology, 18,* 633–638.

Tran, T. V., Fitzpatrick, T. R., Berg, W. R., & Wright, R., Jr. (1996). Acculturation, health, stress, and psychological distress among elderly Hispanics. *Journal of Cross-Cultural Gerontology, 11,* 149–165.

U.S. Census Bureau. (2011). Facts for features. Older Americans month-May 2010. Available at http://www.census.gov/newsroom/releases%20archives/facts%20for_features_special_editions/cb10-ff06.html

Van Cleve, L., Muñoz, C. E., Savedra, M., Riggs, M., Bossert, E., Grant, M., et al. (2012). Symptoms in children with advanced cancer: Child and nurse reports. *Cancer Nursing, 35,* 115–125. doi:10.1097/NCC.0b013e31821aedba

Ward, E., DeSantis, C., Robbins, A., Kohler, B., & Jemal, A. (2014). Childhood and adolescent cancer statistics. *CA: A Cancer Journal for Clinicians, 64,* 83–103.

Welsh, A. L., Sauaia, A., Jacobellis, J., Min, S. J., & Byers, T. (2005). The effect of two church-based interventions on breast cancer screening rates among Medicaid-insured Latinas. *Preventing Chronic Disease*, (4), A07. http://ncbi.nim.nih.gov/pubmed/16164811

Wu, Z. H., Black, S. A., & Markides, K. S. (2001). Prevalence and associated factors of Cancer screening: Why are so many older Mexican American women never screened? *Preventive Medicine, 33*, 268–273.

Yanez, B., Thompson, E. H., & Stanton, A. L. (2011). Quality of life among Latina breast cancer patients: A systematic review of the literature. *Journal of Cancer Survivorship, 5*(2), 191–207. doi:10.1007/s11764-011-0171-0. Epub 2011 Jan 28.

Chapter 4
An Exploration of Latvian Immigrants' Cancer Experience and Implications for Supportive Interventions

Mara L. Leimanis

Introduction

Psychological distress and coping in immigrant populations, as well as those whom have suffered a particular stress is documented from a range of populations and ethnic groups (Cwikel and Rozovski 1998; Aranda and Knight 1997). However, a cancer diagnosis can aggravate preexisting psychological distress and the effects can be trans-generational (Baider et al. 2006; Consedine et al. 2006; Baider et al. 1996b). Past research has addressed the subject of acculturation versus assimilation among immigrant populations (Fitzpatrick 2000). Acculturation as defined by Nasatir (1991) and Belozersky (1991) happens over a long period of time, and can be a very diversified experience (Fitzpatrick 2000). Acculturation includes language skills, familiarity with the host culture, education and generational factors (Fitzpatrick 2000: Tran et al. 1996). Tran states that acculturation is also defined in terms of language skills and education, which are distinct but related (p. 68), "acculturation is a very different experience than assimilation" (Fitzpatrick 2000, p. 67). Assimilation however, is a temporary situation and is defined as a group of people that belong to a minority group but learn to adapt to the ways of the majority culture and whom are able to retain their own culture. In the context of this chapter, it would seem that Latvians are fairly well-acculturated.

The acculturation process has been associated with positive network structures, which can lower depressive symptoms, and may contribute to better overall quality of life (Lim et al. 2008). Research in this area has largely explored the subject of immigrant populations of breast cancer survivors, and ethnic barriers to screening, prevention, and treatments (Andreeva and Pokhrel 2013). The purpose of this chapter was to explore the experience of Latvian-Canadians who are cancer

M.L. Leimanis (✉)
1221 Oxbow Drive, 49333 Middleville, Michigan, USA
e-mail: mara.leimanis@mail.mcgill.ca

T.R. Fitzpatrick (ed.), *Treating Vulnerable Populations of Cancer Survivors: A Biopsychosocial Approach*, DOI 10.1007/978-3-319-32364-0_4

survivors, from the perspective of medical, spiritual, and caregiving, and to explore the topic of interventions and their effects on well-being and quality of life. This is one of the first studies to explore this subject in a small Baltic ethnic group in Canada. It is hoped that this chapter will also provide further information on coping skills, methods of coping, and community supports as they relate to the experience of Latvians with cancer.

Cancer and Emotional Health

A cancer diagnosis can bring an onset of emotions and reactions which can include symptoms of depression and anxiety, intrusive thoughts, and thoughts of avoidance (Jacobsen et al. 1998). Adjusting to a cancer diagnosis may be mediated by a host of preexisting psychosocial factors including, family and community support, past history, and various key factors such as education and marital status (Weisman 1980). Individuals may also experience a cancer diagnosis while having a preexisting level of distress (Zabora et al. 1997). Distress in patients has been associated with poor treatment compliance, (Colleoni et al. 2000; Kennard et al. 2004; DiMatteo et al. 2000), and treatment outcomes, and long-term survival outcomes (Faller et al. 1999; Prieto et al. 2005).

Immigrants and Cancer

Acculturation is a process of cultural change and psychological change that results following the exchange between cultures was described by Sam and Berry (2010, p. 472). At the individual level, changes may occur in daily behaviors, as well as changes in psychological and physical well-being. Cancer patients may experience a certain degree of distress at the onset of a cancer diagnosis; however this can be made less severe in immigrant groups with certain additional supports (Baider et al. 1996a, b). Even before a cancer diagnosis, ethnic groups exhibit various degrees of fear when seeking certain types of screening such as for prostate cancer (Consedine et al. 2006).

Cancer in Latvians

Cancer amongst Latvians living in Europe will fall into regional norms for the disease in terms of incidence, quality of life issues, and access to healthcare (Dzervite et al. 2012). In the immigrant population in Canada, however, additional stressors may affect their disease progression and treatment. This has been identified as a vulnerable population in one report as compared to U.S.-born populations (Deorose et al. 2007). In the results of a cohort study, immigrants from the former Soviet Union revealed a higher overall mortality from non-natural causes (Becher et al. 2007), and that orientation to a new country, change in self-perception and/or family structure, can affect and disable coping strategies. This stress of immigration can in turn exasperate psychiatric disorders while dealing with a disease such as cancer (Baider et al. 1996a, b).

Family, Community Support, and Cancer

Cancer is known to profoundly affect the entire family, and as we know, the family has also been explored in the literature as being a major source of support for cancer survivors (Baider et al. 1996a). In addition, as an extended network to the family, the greater community may serve as a mediator against the negative effects of diagnosis and treatment as well as long-term survival outcomes. Various therapeutic interventions and supports, have been demonstrated to be beneficial (Fitzpatrick and Remmer 2011), defined as family supports, support from caregivers, and/or community supports. In this, the increase in immigration may also play a role in the influence of social supports and networks, as studied in Mexican populations in the United States (Keefe 1980; Sabogal et al. 1987). Community supports might include religious groups (church), cultural activities, choir, artists groups, sports activities, special interest groups, professional and special interest groups, organizations at the local, national and international level, sororities, veterans groups, and others.

Acculturation, therefore, provides a theoretical basis that helps to clarify the relationship between the various interventions and health and well-being of Latvian cancer survivors, as well as their immediate caregivers (Sam and Berry 2010; Baider 2006).

Methodology

Qualitative Research Design and Approach

A one-time questionnaire was used to explore the relationship between supportive interventions and the cancer experience amongst Latvian immigrants. Participants were selected based on purposive sampling (Lugg and Ahmed 2008). This subjective approach to sampling implies that the chosen subjects are knowledgeable about the subject in question; however, no external judgment is provided by the researchers on the typicality of the subjects.

Data

Data was collected between July and September 2014 from individuals who were actively involved in the Latvian community in several Canadian cities. Written consent was obtained and complete anonymity was preserved, if so indicated by the participant. All participants were aware and gave permission for personal statements to be published for research purposes. The information was collected as self-reported questionnaires by e-mail.

Sample

Purposive sampling is defined as meeting certain criteria, which can relate to quality assurance (Patton 2002). The individuals (N = 11) were placed into four groups; those who were cancer survivors (n = 3), those who were cancer caregivers (n = 4), those who were healthcare providers (n = 2), and those who were spiritual caregivers (n = 2). All participants were Canadian citizens and were connected to their Latvian communities, and had travelled to Latvia at least once as adults. The total sample ranged in age from 33 to 77 years, with three males and eight females. All participants had a university education. (Table 1 presents a complete description of the total sample).

Data Collection Procedures

The protocol for the questionnaires included; (a) an opening statement, (b) an introductory research question, and (c) detailed probing questions to follow additional questions. Participants were to limit their responses to a few pages, and were requested to complete the questionnaire within one hour. This negated the influence of the researcher, allowing participants to control their own responses. As a follow-up, the participants were contacted by the researcher by phone, e-mail, in person or through a direct contact and were allotted 2 weeks' time to respond. When necessary, questions were asked to the researcher for clarification and focused on several areas of their experiences, as described below. All four groups (cancer survivors, cancer caregivers, healthcare providers, and spiritual caregivers) underwent the same protocol and the same questions.

Interview Protocol

You have been asked to participate in a small study titled "The Cancer Experience Amongst Latvian Immigrants." This study will involve exploring various aspects of

Table 1 Demographics for total sample of study participants ($N = 11$)

	(n)	%[a]	Mean	[95 % CI]	SD
Age					
33–77			56.9	46.5–67.3	16.4
Gender					
Male	3	27			
Female	8	73			
Education					
University+	11	100			
College or equivalent	0	0			
High School or less	0	0			
Marital status					
Married/common law	6	54			
Divorced/widowed	2	18			
Never married/single	3	27			
Time of birth					
In Latvia (pre-WWII)	4	36			
During or post-WWII	2	18			
First generation Canadian	5	45			
Type of participant					
Cancer survivor	3	(Male 2, Female 1)			
Cancer caregiver	4	(Male 1, Female 3)			
Healthcare provider	2	(Male 0, Female 2)			
Spiritual caregiver	2	(Male 0, Female 2)			
Latvian heritage influenced cancer experience					
Yes	6	55			
No	5	45			

Note [a]Percentages may not add up to 100 % due to missing data

this subject through the eyes of cancer caregivers, cancer survivors, healthcare providers, and spiritual caregivers. The results of the study will be published in a chapter in an academic text book focusing on various interventions, such as family support, community services, physical fitness, and coping mechanisms, and how these interventions may benefit vulnerable populations of cancer survivors. The book will be directed towards oncology professionals working with cancer patients and survivors; such as social workers, nurses, and psychologists. I thank you for your participation and for sharing your story!

1. *Describe your experience as a Latvian-Canadian/Canadian-Latvian (i.e., how are you linked to Latvia).*
2. *Describe your personal cancer experience (as a caregiver, cancer survivor, healthcare provider, spiritual caregiver).*

3. *Describe how being a Latvian-Canadian/Canadian-Latvian influenced your cancer experience.*
4. *Describe what interventions or supports were used and/or influenced your cancer experience (i.e., traditional-, alternative-, complementary-medicines, psychotherapy, vs. family support only, etc.)*

Data Recording

The responses from the interviews were recorded either as hand-written responses, as type-written by respondents, and logged, and/or transcribed in a password protected file within 1 week of receipt of the response. Space was provided following the questionnaire for additional notes if needed. A word processing program (Microsoft Office WordR) was used to backup all of the stored information. The material was reviewed by a second researcher who was impartial to the collection and interview process, in order to maximize the interpretation of the participant's responses. Free-text from open-ended questions revealed themes and provided a working framework for future studies (Corner et al. 2013; Gall et al. 2003), (however, a robust analysis and coding of the data was not performed).

Results

Table 1 indicate that five participants were born pre-World War II, two participants were born during or just after the war, and four participants were first-born generation Canadians. In the first question posed to the participants, they were asked to describe their experience as an immigrant. The responses were organized by the following groups, (cancer survivors, cancer caregivers, healthcare providers and spiritual caregivers) where the majority of participants describe having experiences of acculturation, while preserving a cultural identity.

Results from the questionnaire:

1. *Describe your experience as a Latvian-Canadian/Canadian-Latvian (i.e. how are you linked to Latvia?).*

Cancer Survivors

In the case of the cancer survivors in this study, all three participants were first generation immigrants, having been born in Latvia, and immigrating as children during World War II (WWII).

One person reported, "*My family and I suffered the horrors of the refugee trek, leaving Latvia on Oct. 25th, 1944…We were in Germany, in 1945 when the war ended, and were placed by the Allies in the safety of the Displaced Person (DP) camp. After living for several years in the DP camps, we were fortunate to be allowed to immigrate to Canada on March 29, 1948.*"

Another participant speaks of life post-immigration:

"*It was easy to integrate into a multicultural society such as Canada. I'm accepted as a Latvian-Canadian without prejudice. I was born in Latvia, and I do speak Latvian at home. I do follow our traditions, our culture, and our religion. I have visited Latvia 4 times.*"

Cancer Caregivers

The cancer caregivers were a mix of first generation immigrants and first-born immigrants to Canada. Most of the statements presented, are representative of acculturation.

"*As a Latvian born in Riga, I came to the United States in 1949 from Germany where our family spent 4 years in displaced persons (DP) camps. After marrying in 1970 I came to Montreal. My connections to the Latvian-Canadian community are because of strong family ties, social activities such as choir, sorority, church and cultural events here and elsewhere.*"

Here is the description of a first-born generation Canadian, having integrated her profession with her cultural and familial ties to Latvia.

"*I am linked to Latvia as I was raised in the Montreal Latvian community and spent many extracurricular hours singing in the Latvian Chorale Choir, dancing traditional Latvian dances with the local dance group, and from a very young age to 15 years old. I also attended Latvian school on the weekends. I am currently involved in the Latvian community, as I am writing a fictional screenplay that takes place in Riga, Latvia.*"

Here is the description of the positive effects of cultural ties.

"*My experience has been mostly positive, as I am fortunate to have been exposed to a rich culture and have made many great friends and acquaintances who share the same beliefs and interests as me.*"

Healthcare Providers

Both healthcare providers represent additional examples of their ties to Latvia.

"*I am the daughter of two Latvians who were born during their families' flight from Latvia post-WWII.*"

"*Born in England, I immigrated with Latvian parents to Canada and was quite active in the Latvian community in Toronto. My husband is a Latvian-Canadian and I have taught all my children to speak Latvian.*"

Spiritual Caregivers

Both spiritual caregivers were able to provide additional accounts of their ties to Latvia.

"My mother was born in Latvia during the Second World War and came to Canada as a refugee. Latvian was my first language, and I participated in Latvian Saturday school, Latvian social and cultural events, and spent one year of high school in a Latvian high school in Germany."

Another participant respondent stated:

"I am a first generation Canadian born of displaced persons (DP) who left Latvia at the end of the war and took up refuge in Germany, then making their way to Belgium and then to Canada to fulfill a year's sponsorship. I was brought up in a family where Latvian was my first language and I, along with my siblings attended Latvian schools and church, scouts, and guides as well as participating in a number of other Latvian youth events. In the early years we searched out doctors, dentists, and even banks in which Latvian was spoken, and where I was a part-time employee while going to school."

In summary, it is evident that all accounts indicate that regardless of current residency, or initial birthplace, Latvian remains a major presence in the lives of participants.

2. *Describe your personal cancer experience (as a caregiver, cancer survivor, healthcare provider, spiritual caregiver).*

Cancer Survivors

The cancer survivors give a personal account of their cancer experience.

"I have been a cancer survivor for 16 years, mostly through hormone therapy... the treatment has not affected my professional life, but as any medical treatments have side effects...it could affect your personal life."

In the second account a cancer survivor describes her experience with prevention and screening.

"In having regular mammogram tests, an early diagnosis of a "mis-shapen" cell...a "lesion"...showed the early signs of breast cancer....Dr. "X" performed the surgery...later I received radiation treatment."

Cancer Caregivers

In the case of cancer caregivers, their responses widely varied, in that in some instances only limited care was given in a supportive fashion as described:

"I helped with transportation, accompanied my family to doctor's visits, and was an information gatherer."

Or more acute and personal experiences:

"My mother had been in remission for Non-Hodgkins Lymphoma for several years before the disease came back with a vengeance and went un-diagnosed again until its very late stages before her death in September 2008…my father was suddenly diagnosed with salivary gland cancer a few weeks after my mothers' passing, and after a few short months of care, passed away in January of 2009. My experience was life-changing, and it altered many family relationships in ways I'd never imagined. The entire experience was truly eye-opening and from which I have learned a tremendous deal."

"My mother developed breast cancer that ultimately spread to her liver. My mother decided she was going to heal the cancer herself through natural homeopathic means, and ultimately refused Western medical treatments. Her demands were high as I had to seek out her frequent requests to find the materials she needed for her attempted treatments, and at times, the demands were eccentric and complex. In the end, my experience as a caregiver was a harrowing one, emotionally and physically, and I was not prepared for the demands of this disease and what was required from me as a caregiver."

Additionally, cancer caregivers remark on their information needs, and attempts at seeking psychosocial supports, however with resistance encountered from a cancer survivor:

"As a support partner…I consulted library books and read, to better understand the tests, procedures and medical options…my husband relied heavily on his doctor's advice from the initial diagnosis to the follow-up, which meant that he not only had my support but also encouragement to seek (at a later phase) a second opinion. I have tried to encourage some additional psychological interventions without success."

Healthcare Providers

Interestingly, one healthcare provider remarks on a perspective, not captured by any of the cancer caregivers.

"As a healthcare provider I find cancer care inspiring."

Spiritual Caregivers

From the perspective of spiritual caregivers, there is a more objective overview of the cancer experience, and their demonstrates that caregiver role can differ, from that of the immediate family.

"There are so many different personality styles, ages, forms of cancer, and cultural beliefs, and values in one person's experience of cancer…what is the nature of their fear, resilience, love, survival through someone's cancer experience…it is rare to find a cancer patient who has a lukewarm reaction to the fact they have cancer…the disease often forces them to claim who they are and what they believe in".

"I am not afraid of gently touching people…to gently stroke their arm or face, or even kiss their forehead after having blessed them with the laying on of hands"…"for others I would sing with them or to them."

3. *Describe how being a Latvian-Canadian/Canadian-Latvian influenced your cancer experience.*

This question revealed a dichotomy and wide range of responses, from emotionally charged, to emotionally indifferent. Responses are divided between both positive and negative responses.

Cancer Survivors

Cancer survivors do not attribute their cancer experience as having many cultural or ethnic ties, but remark on the importance of good healthcare.

"*Being a Latvian-Canadian did not have any special significance, only that as a Canadian I received the best care possible to help me deal with breast cancer…I was given the professional care of a psychiatrist…to help me deal with the psychological stress.*"

"*Personally my ethnic background has not influenced my treatment. I have not consulted, religious, psychological or any other support group. Only my immediate family has knowledge of my cancer experience.*"

Cancer Caregivers

The responses of cancer caregivers involve the role of language, community supports as witnessed by some, to be more profound and yet for others, a matter of convenience or lifestyle choices.

"*We often spoke Latvian amongst ourselves during or after the appointment.*"

"*Being a Latvian-Canadian–I was raised in the Latvian-Canadian community. I attended Latvian camp, school, and cultural functions. I was whiteness to, and inherited many quality family values, from my parents and through different relationships with friends and other members of the Latvian-Canadian community. I feel as if I received a tremendous amount of support from the community, which helped in dealing with the events leading up to, at the time of, and after my parents passing.*"

In this recount, the participant comments on feelings of disconnect, shame, and isolation.

"*Latvians are known for their hard workmanship, and this was the way that I was raised in my Latvian-Canadian family…having these qualities influenced my approach, and I was able to remain strong for my mother through her battle. But this hard shell also intervened with connecting emotionally with myself during this process, which I had to reconcile with later on after she passed away. I anticipated my mother would reach out to the Latvian-Canadian community, but instead she shied away from it, perhaps feeling some shame for not being able to face the questions if asked about her decisions regarding her non-Western medical treatment(s). Unfortunately, there was no time for me to reach out to the community for support, and support was not offered. I believe this is also because illness tends to be a private matter in Latvian families, and unless asked to participate, Latvians generally shy away. But on the emotional side of being Latvian, growing up with pagan ideologies and influences in my Latvian upbringing, also made me more open to my mother's Latvian homeopathic remedies and her trying different natural treatments.*"

Issues surrounding community and privacy were revealed by one participant.

"*Individual privacy is partly a personality trait of many Latvians, but disclosure of cancer seems to be more private than that of other illnesses. Perhaps this is because cancer often requires long-term care. Among men especially there exists the unwillingness to see support groups. Many shy away from disclosure regarding cancer, but even heart surgery is revealed more easily, probably the type of cancer also influences the privacy issue.*"

Healthcare Providers

The view of a healthcare provider is summarized very briefly, and states that nationality does not influence the cancer experience.

"*People either catastrophize the diagnosis or embrace it, but most eventually accept it. This does not depend upon their nationality.*"

Spiritual Caregivers

From the perspective of spiritual caregivers, a commentary describing both the private experience and the community experience.

"*I would listen to peoples' stories of youth and deportation, immigration journeys, and incorporate them in the funeral services….the whole community was involved in their grief.*"

"*I found that my family and relatives behaved in very private, rational ways to cancer. The disease was not talked about in detail, and revealing emotions was not part of discussions except in one rare conversation…Cancer was seen as a problem to solve…and there was an attitude of "pull yourself up by the bootstraps",… relatives engaged in a sense of disbelief and denial of the immensity of a terminal case of cancer.*"

4. *Describe what interventions or supports were used and/or influenced your cancer experience (i.e., traditional-, alternative-, complementary-medicines, psychotherapy, family support only, etc.).*

Cancer Survivors

The comments from the cancer survivors reveal the use of traditional medical interventions, as well as family support:

"I am grateful to everyone for their care in dealing with my breast cancer, so that I am able to say I am "cancer free" for 7 years."

"My cancer experience was very traditional...from my general practitioner to my urologist, to surgery to hormone therapy, I never sought any counseling or support, except for family...a book about the influence of the subconscious mind which I believed in, helped to strengthen my resolve to get well."

Cancer Caregivers

In the case of cancer caregivers, there is insight into collusion and various forms of coping.

"In most cases traditional treatment methods have been used (chemotherapy, radiation, drugs), and the cancer survivor has not been interested in complementary medicines, or possible "cures" using diet, meditation or exercise...perhaps coming from a conservative background that makes "alternatives" an unfamiliar choice...the cancer survivor wants to follow what the doctor says, and put trust in them, rather than look elsewhere...it is easier not to question things too much."

"I was fortunate to have a close circle of friends who were able to provide some comfort and support, during this tragic and unfortunate time—of which many of were able to relate, empathize and share from their own experiences."

"Our experience relied chiefly on traditional medicine and rapid response to the diagnosis. Following the biopsy and necessary surgery, trust was almost entirely placed in the doctor's experience and expertise in regards to the medication. My husband turned to some other supports when his sister developed breast and later ovarian cancer. She was part of a cancer support group at the Princess Margaret in Toronto. This meditation and laughter therapy was intended to relieve some of the stress of chemotherapy and worry about the illness. At the time he read a book on the subconscious mind. He has not been interested in any other active therapy-whether exercise or psychological. My own understanding is that meditation can play a strong role in recovery along with traditional treatments."

Another respondent stated:

"As my mother was using natural Latvian medicinal treatments, that her mother had taught her to use (for other ailments, not cancer) and that she had read about. I was supportive of her trying these traditional methods, as she had made a concerted decision to do so (i.e. placing a cabbage leaf over her breast, using Latvian herbs, keeping amber stones in her hands/on her body). These traditional Latvian methods did influence my experience positively as it instilled hope, but other family members and Latvian community members thought the methods were based on

myths, and were carried out with poor judgment. She new she would be criticized for her decision-making from some people in the Latvian community, as she had been following healing methods from Satya Sai Baba, a controversial Indian guru and spiritual leader. I believe she obtained much emotional peace by taking this path, and I was supportive of her as she dabbled in this community, knowing it made her feel good. Six months before she passed away, I looked to psychotherapy one-two times a week to get me through this arduous process and time period. I continued with it a year after my mother passed, to help make sense of what I had just gone through. Also, traditional Chinese massages (deep tissue and shiatsu) helped me cope with the stress of this time and human touch helped me to connect emotionally. My sister and I were each other's rocks to lean on, but as we were on our own, looking back, I wish we could have asked our community and family to be more involved in order to help us emotionally."

Healthcare Providers

The one healthcare provider revealed that the primary source of support is family:

"*All available supports are important but I have found that a supportive, caring family is the most significant one, enabling adjustment to the diagnosis and for moving forward.*"

Spiritual Caregivers

The spiritual caregivers commented on the diversity of treatments and how collusion affected their own coping skills.

"*My personal experience with cancer with my relatives strongly influenced me to learn how to support patients by providing psychotherapeutic and spiritual support. I felt my family lacked the resources to effectively discuss, support and grow from their cancer experience as a larger group…I wished to learn what I did not learn in my family structure in order to be attentive to others, who are managing sometimes terminal diseases. I wanted to play a more active role in asking questions, sharing my experience, advocating for, and supporting family members and others struggling with cancer.*"

Various supports sought by participants is summarized in Table 2. This includes seeking medical, and family supports.

Table 2 Summary of treatments and supports sought by various Latvian groups interviewed ($N = 11$)

Groups	HP (%)	CS (%)	SC (%)	CC (%)
Medical treatments				
Traditional (Western)	1 (50 %)	3 (100 %)	1 (50 %)	2 (50 %)
Chemotherapy		1 50 %)		
Radiotherapy		2 (66 %)		
Hormone therapy		1 (33 %)		
Surgery		2 (66 %)		
Non-traditional (homeopathic)			1 (50 %)	2 (50 %)
Prevention and long-term follow-up		1 (33%)		1 (25 %)
Exercise		1 (33 %)		
Massage (deep tissue)				1 (25 %)
Diet		2 (66 %)		
Supplements (vitamins)		1 (33 %)		
Healthy environment		1 (33%)		
Meditation		1 (33 %)		1 (25%)
Supports				
Transportation				1 (25 %)
Information seeking				2 (50%)
Education				1 (25%)
Family support	1 (50 %)	2 (66 %)	2 (100 %)	4 (100 %)
Community support			1 (50 %)	1 (25 %)
Psychosocial intervention	1 (50 %)	1 (33 %)		1 (25 %)
Psychotherapy		2 (66 %)	1 (50 %)	1 (25 %)
Subconsious mind		1 (33 %)		
Positive thinking		1 (33 %)		1 (25 %)
Spiritual support			2 (100 %)	

Note HP-healthcare provider; *CS*-cancer survivor; *SC*-spiritual caregiver; *CC*-cancer caregiver

Discussion

This preliminary exploration of Latvian immigrants' cancer experience and implications for supportive care, revealed that the majority of our respondents experience acculturation and are eventually assimilated into the dominant culture. Together with this, there was some degree of collusion felt by first-born generation Canadian-Latvians, who expressed that the need for privacy, and secrecy, was necessary for those affected by cancer. The family was revealed as the major source of support by nearly all participants—nine (82 %) in total as seen in Table 2.

Latvian immigrant cancer survivors are a vulnerable population for whom culturally tailored cancer care programs are needed, as has been provided to other immigrant and minority groups (Howard et al. 2007; Chiu 2001). However, it has been shown that knowledge of the English language and resilience can lower depressive scores, and help to ease the post migration transition period, as found for mid-life woman from the former Soviet Union (Miller and Chandler 2002). In Balneaves et al. (2007), Punjabi woman with a breast cancer diagnosis describe stress factors that may be negated by family supports, indicating the need for family-centered models of care (Balneaves et al. 2007). Together, this suggests that immigrants, who undergo acculturation, require additional attention and supports, as compared to their fully assimilated counterparts.

It has been shown that cancer preventative behaviors for Eastern European immigrant woman, are fairly consistent, regardless of the host country, access to healthcare, or education level. A total of 30 studies from 1996 to 2013 reveal that Eastern European woman under-utilize breast cancer screening options, in part, due to insufficient knowledge about early detection and an external locus of control. In that, their decision-making process, regarding personal health matters, was caused by uncontrollable factors (such as the environment, other people, or a higher power) (Andreeva and Pokhrel 2013). This under-screening and inadequate engagement in health prevention could also be applied to other diseases or conditions as well.

Collusion is also highlighted as one major theme from the participant responses, which is generally defined as a secret agreement between two or more people who are trying to deceive persons in the immediate circle of contacts (e.g., a doctor and patient withholding information from the patients' children) (Oxford 1990). In the case of health and healthcare, any information regarding a diagnosis, prognosis, and medical details, can be withheld from friends or familys involved, with the care of the patient, whereby in the case of a terminal illness, news is withheld from the patients' children, or primary caregivers. It has been a phenomenon observed in both Western and non-Western societies that most commonly center around recurrence, deterioration, and palliative treatments (NCI 2009). In our narratives, it appears as though the collusion may be partial or complete. As some participants mentioned the need to maintain secrecy regarding the illness from the community, which resulted in feelings of isolation, shame, and loneliness. In cases where participants were able to reveal the diagnosis with immediate friends and family, the support resources were more abundant and helpful.

Spiritual resources have been revealed as a key theme among Chinese immigrants with breast cancer in the USA along with family closeness, alternative therapy, art, prose and literature, and culture-specific support groups (Chiu 2001). In the population sampled for the purpose of this study, religion and spirituality was not highlighted as a major theme.

Implications for Clinical Practice

Caregivers, and children of first generation Latvians (i.e., first-born generation Canadian-Latvians), in some cases considered their ethnicity as a hindrance in their personal coping mechanisms, and highlighted either partial or complete collusion in the family structure. Cancer survivors comment on the benefits of positive thinking, lifestyle choices and non-traditional treatments (natural). Immigrants who undergo the process of acculturation, require additional attention and supports, as compared to their assimilated counterparts. Special attention is required from healthcare providers to address the needs of this vulnerable population, especially in regards to education and language instruction where needed. Healthcare practitioners should therefore, reach out to family members to stress the importance of early screening and treatment for their relative(s) with cancer language.

Several limitations of the study are warranted. Only Latvian immigrants and Canadian-Latvians supplied the study sample and the sample size was limited in number and to those that agreed to participate. Many did not want to participate commenting: "I have nothing to say" as Latvians tend to be private in nature, and present a form of a closed community, one that can be found in other Northern European cultures (Lanier 2000, p. 55). Implications for future research include the need to further explore the subject with a broader sampling size, given the inherent heterogeneity (age, cancer type, profession, gender, and ties and links to Latvia, i.e., those of birthplace of Latvia versus first-born generation Canadians) as in such a defined and small population. Additionally, a more robust experimental design could be utilized.

In summary, the practitioner in a clinical oncology setting must recognize the family dynamics, and that there may be issues surrounding privacy for the patient, collusion between family members on the severity and gravity of the disease, as well as that the primary support system for the patient, falls to the children and immediate family. As a first step, supports within the community should be explored, as physical health referrals within the hospital system may not satisfy the families need for "keeping it in the family." Rather, the immediate caregivers should be targeted as recipients of additional supports.

Acknowledgements The author would like to thank all of the participants for their contributions. Dr. Leimanis is supported by The Latvian National Federal of Canada (LNFC), and the Council of Montreal Latvian Organizations (CMLO).

References

Andreeva, V. A., & Pokhrel, P. (2013). Breast cancer screening utilization among Eastern European immigrant women worldwide: A systematic literature review and a focus on psychological barrriers. *Psycho-Oncology, 22*(12), 2664–2675.

Aranda, M. P., & Knight, B. G. I. (1997). The influence of ethnicity and culture on the caregiver stress and coping process: A Sociocultural review and analysis. *The Gerontologist, 37*(3), 342–354.

Baider, L., Peretz, T., & Kaplan De-Nour, A. (1992). Effect of the holocaust on coping with cancer. *Social Science and Medicine, 34*(1), 11–15.

Baider, L., Cooper, C. L., Kaplan De-Nour, A. (Eds.). (1996a). *Cancer and the Family*. Oxford, England: John Wiley & Sons Chichester.

Baider, L., Kaufman, B., Ever-Hadani, P., & DeNour, A. K. (1996b). Coping with additional stresses: comparative study of healthy and cancer patient new immigrants. *Social Science and Medicine, 42*, 1077–1084.

Baider, L., Goldzweig, B. L., Ever-Hadani, P., & Peretz, T. (2006). Psychological distress and coping in breast cancer patients and healthy women whose parents survived the Holocaust. *Psycho-Oncology, 15*(7), 635–646.

Balneaves, L. G., Bottorff, J. L., Grewal, S. K., Paromita, N., Johnson, J. L., & Howard, A. F. (2007). Family support of immigrant Punjabi woman with breast cancer. *Family & Community Health, 30*(1), 16–28.

Becher, H., Razum, O., Kyobutungi, C., Laki, J., Ott, J. J., Ronellenfitsch, U., & Winkler, V. (2007). Mortality of Immigrants from the Former Soviet Union: Results of a cohort study. *Deutsches Ärzteblatt,* 104(23): A1655–A1661.

Belozersky, I. (1991). *Therapeutic interventions with Soviet refugee families.* Boston, MA: Paper presented at the Jewish Family and Children's Services.

Chiu, L. (2001). Spiritual resources of Chinese immigrants with breast cancer in the USA. *International Journal of Nursing Studies, 38*(2), 175–184.

Colleoni, M., Mandala, M., Peruzzotti, G., Robertson, C., Bredart, A., & Goldhirsch, A. (2000). Depression and degree of acceptance of adjuvant cytotoxic drugs. *Lancet, 356*(9238), 1326–1327. doi:10.1016/S0140-6736(00)02821-X. S0140-6736(00)02821-X [pii].

Consedine, N. S., Morgenstern, A. H., Kudadjie-Gyamfi, E., Magai, C., & Neugut, A. I. (2006). Prostate cancer screening behavior in men from seven ethnic groups: The fear factor. *Cancer Epidemiology, Biomarkers and Prevention, 15*(2), 228–237.

Corner, J., Wagland, R., Glaser, A., & Richards, M. (2013). Qualitative analysis of patients' feedback from a PROMs survey of cancer patients in England. *BMJ Open, 3*, e002316. doi:10.1136/bmjopen-2012-002316

Cwikel, J., & Rozovski, U. (1998). Coping with the Stress of Immigration among New Immigrants to Isreal from Commonwealth of Independent States (CiS) who were Exposed to Chernobyl: The Effect of Age. *The International Journal of Aging and Human Development, 46*(4), 305–318.

Deorose, K. P., Escarce, J. J., & Lurie, N. (2007). Immigrants and health care: Sources of vulnerability. *Health Affairs, 26*(5), 1258–1268.

DiMatteo, M. R., Lepper, H. S., & Croghan, T. W. (2000). Depression is a risk factor for noncompliance with medical treatment: meta-analysis of the effects of anxiety and depression on patient adherence. *Archives of Internal Medicine, 160*(14), 2101–2107. ioi90679[pii].

Dzervite, A., Pranka, M., Lace, T., Rungule, R., Miklasevics, E., & Gardovskis, J. (2012). Key factors contributing to quality of life for breast cancer patients in Latvia: Supplementing quantitative surveys with qualitative interviews. *Acta Chirurgica Latviensis, 12*, 3–10.

Faller, H., Bulzebruck, H., Drings, P., & Lang, H. (1999). Coping, distress, and survival among patients with lung cancer. *Archives of General Psychiatry, 56*(8), 756–762.

Fitzpatrick, T. (2000). Elderly Russian Jewish Immigrants. In S. Aleman, T. Fitzpatrick, T.V. Tran, & E.W. Gonzalez (Eds.), *Therapeutic interventions with ethnic elders, health and social issues* (pp. 55–78). New York: The Haworth Press.

Fitzpatrick, T. R., & Remmer, J. (2011). Needs, expectation and attendance among participants of a cancer wellness centre in Montreal, Quebec. *Journal of Cancer Survivorship, 5*, 235–246.

Gall, M. D., Gall, J. P., & Borg, W. R. (2003). *Educational research: An introduction* (7th ed.). Boston, MA: A&B Publications.

Howard, A. F., Bottorff, J. L., Balneaves, L. G., & Grewal, S. K. (2007). Punjabi Immigrant Women's Breast Cancer Stories. *Journal of Immigrant Minority Health., 9*, 269–279.

Jacobsen, P. B., Widows, M. R., Hann, D. M., Andrykowski, M. A., Kronish, L. E., & Fields, K. K. (1998). Posttraumatic stress disorder symptoms after bone marrow transplantation for breast cancer. *Psychosomatic Medicine, 60*(3), 366–371.

Keefe, S. E. (1980). Acculturation and the extended family among urban Mexican Americans. In A. M. Padilla (Ed.), *Acculturation: Theory, models, and some new findings* (pp. 85–110). Boulder, CO: Westview Press.

Kennard, B. D., Stewart, S. M., Olvera, R., Bawdon, R. E., Oh Ailin, A., Lewis, C. P., & Winick, N. J. (2004). Nonadherence in adolescent oncology patients: preliminary data on psychological risk factors and relationships to outcome. *Journal of Clinical Psychology in Medical Settings, 11*(1), 31–39. doi:10.1023/B:JOCS.0000016267.21912.74

Lanier, S. A. (2000). *Foreign to Familiar: A Guide to Understanding Hot- and Cold-Climate Cultures*. Hagerstown, MD: McDougall Publisher.

Lim, J. W., Yi, J., & Zebrack, B. (2008). Acculturation, social support, and quality of life for Korean immigrant breast and gynecological cancer survivors. *Ethnicity & Health, 13*(3), 243–260.

Lugg, G. R., & Ahmed, H. A. (2008). Nurses perception of methicillin-resistant *Staphylococcus aureus*: Impacts on practice. *British Journal of Infection Control, 9*(1), 8–14.

Miller, A. M., & Chandler, P. J. (2002). Acculturation, Resilience, and Depression in Midlife Women from the Former Soviet Union. *Nursing Research,* 51(1), 26-32.

Nasatir, S. B. (1991, May). *The challenge of Jewish acculturation and integration*. The paper presented at the Integration and Acculturation of Soviet Jewish Immigrants Professional Conference, Chicago, IL.

National Cancer Institute. Communication in cancer care (PDQ): Health professional version [retrieved on 20 Apr 2009]. Available from http://www.cancer.gov/cancertopics/pdq/supportivecare/communication/HealthProfessional

Oxford Dictionary. 2nd edn (1990). New York: Oxford Press.

Patton, M. Q. (2002). Qualitative evaluation and research methods (3rd ed.). Newbury Park, CA: Sage.

Prieto, J. M., Atala, J., Blanch, J., Carreras, E., Rovira, M., Cirera, E., et al. (2005). Role of depression as a predictor of mortality among cancer patients after stem-cell transplantation. *Journal of Clinical Oncology, 23*(25), 6063–6071. doi:10.1200/JCO.2005.05.751. JCO.2005.05.751[pii].

Sabogal, F., Marin, G., Otero-Sabogal, R., Marin, B. V. O., & Perez-Stable, E. J. (1987). Hispanic familism and acculturation: What changes and what doesn't? *Hispanic Journal of Behavioural Sciences, 9*, 397–412.

Sam, D. L., & Berry, J. W. (2010). Acculturation When individuals and groups of different cultural backgrounds meet. *Perspectives on Psychological Science, 5*(4), 472–481. doi:10.1177/1745691610373075

Tran, T. V., Fitzpatrick, T. R., Berg, W. R., & Wright, R. Jr. (1996). Acculturation, health, stress, and psychological distress among elderly Hispanics. *Journal of Cross-Cultural Gerontology*, 11, 149–165.

Weisman, A. D., Worden, J. W., & Sobel, H. J. (1980). Psychosocial screening and interventions with cancer patients: A research report. Bethesda, MD: National Cancer Institute.

Zabora, J., Blanchard, C. G., Smith, E. D., Roberts, C. S., Glajchcn, M., Sharp, J. W., et al. (1997). Prevalence of psychological distress among cancer patients across the disease continuum. *Journal of Psychosocial Oncology, 15*(2), 73–87.

Chapter 5
Survivorship Issues Among Muslim Women with Cancer

Suzanne Y. Bushfield

The purpose of this chapter is to examine survivorship issues among the diverse population of Muslim women living in the United States, and to describe culturally competent strategies for intervention that are sensitive to the needs of Muslim women facing breast cancer.

Introduction

Breast Cancer Prevalence in the U.S.

One in 8 women in the U.S. can expect to be diagnosed with breast cancer during her lifetime (Centers for Disease Control 2015). It is the most common cancer in women worldwide, and the second leading cause of death for women in the U.S. (CDC 2015). In the United States, 220,000 women are diagnosed with breast cancer each year. Despite progress in detection and treatment, breast cancer is still a killer: over 40,000 women die of breast cancer each year (CDC 2015).

Survivorship

Breast cancer mortality rates have been declining since 1990 (CDC 2015). As overall death rates from breast cancer decline, surviving breast cancer is a reality for increasing numbers of women. With nearly 14 million cancer survivors in the United States, women make up 54 % of cancer survivors (National Cancer Institute

S.Y. Bushfield (✉)
Arizona State University, 3805 S. Mesquite Ave., Sioux Falls, SD 57110, USA
e-mail: Suzanne.bushfield2@gmail.com

T.R. Fitzpatrick (ed.), *Treating Vulnerable Populations of Cancer Survivors: A Biopsychosocial Approach*, DOI 10.1007/978-3-319-32364-0_5

2014). Among cancer survivors, the largest group is survivors of breast cancer, who make up 22 % of all cancer survivors. Women with early stage breast cancer may now expect to survive 5 years or more. Women who survive breast cancer have benefitted from two key factors: early detection and improved treatment (CDC 2015). Early detection, through breast cancer screening, is known to significantly reduce mortality (Cedolini 2014). As cancer death rates continue to decline among women, attention to survivorship concerns have grown. Survivors of breast cancer often experience a number of health challenges, including pain, fatigue, cognitive changes (Fitzpatrick et al. 2012), swelling, weight loss or gain, sexual dysfunction, as well as fear of recurrence (National Cancer Institute 2014). This fear is not unfounded: even though early detection and effective treatments have improved breast cancer survivorship, the risk of relapse or recurrence persists even 15 years after initial diagnosis (Natarajan et al. 2009).

Muslim Women in America

Muslim communities in America may differ sharply from those in other countries. The population of Muslims in America is diverse. Some 35 % of American Muslims are descendants of African slaves. Arab Muslims make up nearly 30 % of the population in the U.S., and South Asians, 25 % (Haddad 2006). Other Muslim immigrant groups have assimilated in differing degrees. Some 7 million people among the diverse groups of Muslims in America adhere to Islamic guidance on matters of both public and private life (Haddad 2006).

Cultural and religious factors have a strong influence on health behaviors and gender roles (Lum 2003; Miller and Thoresen 2003). Yet, practitioners often view Muslims in America according to prevailing, and often negative, cultural norms (Bushfield and Fitzpatrick 2010; Hodge and Bushfield 2006). Religion and culture may therefore have a particularly significant impact on Muslim women and their health care (Matin and LeBaron 2004). The degree of religiosity, and adherence to tenets of Islam may differ among American Muslim women, but issues related to modesty, the role of women in the family and putting others' needs ahead of her own, and the importance of family involvement in health care decisions have contributed to barriers in health care for Muslim women in America (Matin and LeBaron 2004; Rashidi and Rajaram 2000; Morioka-Douglas et al. 2004). These barriers are significant in understanding health disparities, and the particular needs of Muslim women in America who are diagnosed with, and survive, breast cancer.

Literature Review

Cancer Demographics and Health Disparities

Health disparities have different health outcomes among groups. Disparities may occur both in disease prevalence and death rates. While causes of health disparities may be unknown, considerable research is directed toward a better understanding of the variety of factors that contribute to different outcomes.

Health disparities in cancer have been found based on race, ethnicity, gender, immigrant status, education, geography, and income (CDC 2012). For example, black women have a lower incidence rate of breast cancer, yet have a 41 % higher mortality rate (CDC 2012). Geographic inequalities due to remoteness, and socioeconomic disadvantage have been identified (Dasgupta et al. 2012). For women in rural communities or without proximity to regional cancer centers, disparities may be magnified (Peek and Han 2004). Early detection is a key factor in improved outcomes, yet minorities are less likely to participate in screening activities (Taplin et al. 2012). Cancers undetected through breast cancer screening are often assumed to have a poorer prognosis (Coldman and Phillips 2014). The type of cancer diagnosed may also influence outcomes. Black women have more frequent diagnoses of cancer types that have fewer treatment options (Agurs-Collins et al. 2010). The timeliness of follow-up care is also important. Longer intervals between initial diagnosis and treatment results in poorer outcomes (Olivetto et al. 2002; Jones et al. 2005), and women in rural areas, those with lower incomes, and minorities are among those with long intervals between diagnosis and treatment. Treatment advances have been significant with breast cancer. Yet the quality of treatment received may differ for minority groups (Lund et al. 2008).

Survivorship and Health Disparities

Health disparities have received considerable research and policy attention, leading to interventions aimed at increasing culturally appropriate efforts to increase access and reduce barriers, in order to improve survivorship. Increased participation in mammography screening, leading to early detection, has contributed significantly to the nearly 20 % decline in breast cancer in the recent past. (Padela et al. 2015). However, women from racial and ethnic minorities have been known to participate less in screening activities and therefore may not see the benefits of screening and resulting improvement in survivorship. Overall trends of screening mammography among American Muslim women remain illusive (Padela et al. 2015) since there are no population-based repeated surveys. Additionally, culturally adapted breast cancer screening for Muslim women is not generally available (Hasnain et al. 2014), and may contribute to the lack of participation by Muslim women. While white women are more often diagnosed with breast cancer, minority women have a higher mortality rate and more challenges for survivorship. The survival rate also drops considerably when comorbidities are present. Significantly, high blood pressure, osteoporosis, and heart disease as comorbidities can double the mortality rate from breast cancer. (Kohler et al. 2015). These comorbidities are also subject to racial and ethnic disparities. Variations in outcomes are reflected in health data which indicate all ethnic groups have lower survival rates than white women, and Black African and South Asian women have lower survival rates due in part to the lack of early detection and the prevalence of health comorbidities (Jack et al. 2009).

Other issues have been found to have an impact on survivorship. Economic burden and fear of re-occurrence have been found to have a significant impact (American Cancer Society 2015). Survivorship care plans are intended to address the holistic needs and concerns for breast cancer survivors, such as recognizing emotions, accepting fears, reducing stress, staying well informed, receiving follow-up health care, making healthy choices, and nurturing strong support systems (American Cancer Society 2015). These survivorship care plans may also need to address the specific cultural and family needs of Muslim women, recognizing the differences among Muslim women.

Health Challenges for Survivors

Breast cancer survivors have described a variety of health challenges that impact quality of life. Chief among these are fatigue, pain, sexual dysfunction, swelling, and sleep disturbance, cognitive changes, nerve damage, weight loss or gain, dental and mouth problems, and depression (CDC 2015). For survivors who have lived through the challenge of breast cancer, some, none, or all of these concerns may be experienced. The personal experience of each person will differ, and the individualized nature of being a cancer survivor should be acknowledged (Hebdon et al. 2015).

Other issues have been found to have an impact on survivorship. Economic burden and fear of re-occurrence have been found to have a significant impact (Am Ca Soc 2015). The shift from understanding breast cancer as an acute illness to recognizing it as a chronic disease, with long term consequences that may be both positive and negative, represents a paradigm shift in health care (Hebdon et al. 2015). Survivorship care plans are intended to address the holistic needs and concerns for breast cancer survivors, such as recognizing emotions, accepting fears, reducing stress, staying well informed, follow-up health care, making healthy choices, and strong support systems (Am Ca Soc 2015).

Social Support

The transition from patient to survivor is a challenge to women who have faced breast cancer. Some women do not wish to identify themselves as survivors, and reject the term "survivor" (Hebdon et al. 2015). Nevertheless, they acknowledge the importance of support in a variety of ways, not limited to traditional support groups (Morris et al. 2014). African American women have expressed the importance of social support from peers and family, and particularly the need for support from other African American women who have experienced breast cancer (Mollica and Nemeth 2015). Many Muslim women in America are socially and linguistically isolated, and therefore may need social support through small groups within their cultural groups, and with recognition for the gatekeeping role of men as heads of households (Shirazi et al. 2013).

Fear and Relapse

Adapting to, and surviving from, cancer may be a lifelong process of reappraisal and adjustment over time (Naus et al. 2009). Due to the long trajectory of cancer survivorship for some, fear of recurrence may be both a long term and realistic concern. The centrality of cancer survivorship in one's self concept has been linked both to engaging in behaviors to support well-being, and with greater psychological distress (Helgeson 2011). The latter was present when the central concept of being a cancer survivor was present, and when cancer was viewed in more negative terms. Some 83 % of cancer survivors identify themselves as "survivors" as opposed to "patients" or "victims" (Park et al. 2009). Uncertainty during the transition from patient to survivor is very common during active treatment for cancer (Garofalo et al. 2009).

Spiritual Needs

Isolation and loneliness are common among women who have experienced breast cancer (Rosedale 2009). This isolation may be a function of awareness of mortality and the existential threat of breast cancer. The heightened distress experienced by survivors, including survival guilt, may have a spiritual dimension (Maxwell and Aldredge-Clanton 1994).

Muslim Women in America

Religious barriers are not well understood. In addition to the well-documented health disparities experienced by minority women, religious differences may play a significant role. For Muslims who follow Shari'a law, increasingly under legal scrutiny in the U.S., there may be further tensions. Unlike legal systems in the U.S., Shari'a law governs public behavior, private behavior, and private beliefs (Hodge and Bushfield 2006).

Islam includes five main pillars of faith: (1) testimony that Allah is the one true god; (2) prayer, conducted five times daily at dawn, noon, mid afternoon, sunset, and night; (3) giving support to the needy; (4) fasting during Ramadan; and (5) the annual pilgrimage to Mecca (Hodge 2005). Reliance on Shari'a law and practice of the main tenets of faith for Muslims reflect both the saliency of religion in their individual lives, as well as the degree of acculturation (Hodge 2005). Current political tensions all have an impact on Muslim women in America.

Muslim women differ considerably in a variety of experiences as to the role of women in their distinct communities. Traditionalism and acculturation are both important factors in understanding the specific impact of religion on Muslim women (Salman 2012). Nevertheless, Muslim women have a number of challenges when accessing health care in the United States. Religious beliefs and cultural differences influence Muslim women's choices in participation and follow up in cancer screening and care (Rashidi and Rajaram 2000). Modesty, perceived discrimination in health care, fatalism, cancer knowledge and awareness, family involvement, and role of women in the family have been found to have an influence on Muslim women seeking health care in the U.S. (Matin and LeBaron 2004). These factors may serve to prevent women from seeking treatment or delaying treatment for breast cancer, thereby impeding survivorship. Nearly all American Muslims report lower rates of mammography (less than the 67 % national average for all women). Muslim women participate in rates lower than 60 % (Grabler et al. 2012; Padela and Curlin 2013).

While religious barriers are not well understood, religious values may influence health behaviors in different ways than socioeconomic or acculturative factors. When viewed in context, household duties, and responsibilities for family caregiving, in the context of Muslim women, may be viewed not just as a role, but as part of one's duty to Allah. For many Muslim women, the fear of being a burden due to illness is a strong influence on health behavior. In the family context, dependency for transportation, financial support, and reliance on the male (father or husband) as the decision maker may prevent access to health care. Muslim women may also fear public discrimination in the health care system. Some Muslim women may see illness as dishonorable, or punishment from Allah for past sins. This more fatalistic view may also influence health care outcomes and survivorship for women with breast cancer.

Religion-Related Factors

In 2001, some 1200 studies were found to have quantitatively examined various aspects of religiosity (Koenig and Bussing 2010). Religiosity is a complex construct, and may be described as extrinsic (such as attending public religious meetings) or intrinsic (such as spending time in private religious activities such as prayer, meditation, and study) (Koenig and Bussing 2010). The subjective or intrinsic beliefs are thought to be a more accurate reflection of a person's religiosity (Koenig et al. 2011). Religious attendance and participation in group activities has been related to more social support and better physical health (Salman 2012; Koenig et al. 2011). But it is also related to lower health service use, which may influence survivorship and follow up care. A belief in the presence of the Divine, or religion, carries over into all other dealings (Koenig and Bussing 2010).

The importance of assessing the saliency of religion or worldview in one's life is fundamental to addressing the spiritual needs of others (Hodge and Bushfield 2006). The need for measures, which are more subtle than broad based has been identified (Koenig and Bussing 2010). Spiritual competence, as an aspect of holistic treatment, should be viewed as an active, ongoing process characterized by three ongoing and interrelated dimensions: growing awareness of one's spiritual world view and associated assumptions, limitations and biases; a developing empathic understanding of other's spiritual worldview that is devoid of judgment; and an increasing ability to design and implement appropriate, relevant, interventions that are sensitive to others' world view (Hodge and Bushfield 2006).

Theoretical Perspectives

A multidimensional contextual framework is useful for both understanding and intervening with Muslim women with breast cancer. As a framework for understanding ethnicity, gender, religiosity, immigrant status, economic status, education, and social, political, and environmental factors, a multidimensional contextual framework provides a holistic view of people and their internal and external exchanges (Guadalupe and Lum 2005). This theoretical framework has practice implications that support individual well-being, and active processes with human commonalities, differences, and complexities (Guadalupe and Lum 2005).

Discussion of Implications for Treatment

Holistic treatment aimed at improving survivorship among Muslim women with breast cancer must be culturally sensitive. Culturally appropriate interventions are needed, for example, directed toward Muslim immigrant women who have been found to have low levels of knowledge and awareness of breast cancer and low utilization rates of early detection services. Recognizing the unique social, cultural, and religious dynamics of Muslim women is necessary to develop community based interventions within the diverse Muslim communities in the United States (Shirazi et al. 2013).

Services, which address the special needs of Muslim women for gender specific spaces rather than mixed groups for support, and chemotherapy or mammography, in order to address needs for modesty are critical. Muslim women have identified a preference for gender concordant care, based on religious values of modesty and privacy. Additionally, availability of Halal food, seen as health promoting, and access to a neutral prayer space that is both private and secure are needed. These elements contribute to the positive aspects of Muslim community preference for health care (Padela and Curlin 2012). Opportunities to assess the religious needs related to special dietary needs, hand washing and other practices, and private prayer space may enhance the use of ongoing cancer care for Muslim women and improve outcomes. Opportunities for support from family and community are necessary to address the perception of discrimination toward Muslim women in health care.

Competent Cross-Cultural Practice

Within Muslim communities, women facing breast cancer and other serious illnesses have communicated three distinct themes related to their needs. The first is the dependence created through the illness experience. For some Muslim women, this dependency is associated with feelings of shame and burden, as roles in the family are impacted by illness (Zeilani and Seymour 2012). Family support is seen as critical to address social needs during illness. The individual's religious norms and beliefs are seen as central to one's understanding of illness (Zeilani and Seymour 2012).

A variety of cross-cultural curative factors (Harper-Dorton and Lantz 2007) have been identified which provide additional direction for appropriate interventions addressed at survivorship for Muslim women. These interventions are significant across cultures. Respect for one's worldview may be communicated in attending to the specific needs of Muslim women. Hope may be communicated through the provision of competent services with warmth, kindness, and integrity. Empowering Muslim women, within the context of their own needs, may require adaptation and inclusion of key support people. Cleansing rituals, as an aspect of healing, may carry particular significance for Muslim women. Existential realization may be addressed through making or creating new meaning of the illness trajectory through survivorship, addressing reappraisal of a fatalistic or "punishing Allah" to a more positive religious coping characterized by "Be patient, rely on Allah, and Allah's decrees as a means to cure" (Padela et al. 2015).

Many Muslims in America experienced post-9/11 discrimination since 2001. Negative images of Muslims in the U.S. and elsewhere have led to anti-Muslim sentiment in public life. Muslim women must cope with these expressions of fear and hatred, and their religious identities are challenged in different ways. Some Muslim women have created their own groups through which they challenge existing stereotypes. Others have become more segregated within their Muslim communities, and avoid participation in non-Muslim groups (Bushfield and Fitzpatrick 2010; Haddad 2006). It is therefore particularly important to address the need for improved breast cancer survivorship through culturally sensitive interventions, which may improve access and reduce perceived discrimination.

Conclusions

Muslim women in America have a tendency to not participate in screening activities; they may perceive discrimination from health care providers or have other cultural and religious factors, as well as socioeconomic barriers, to receiving early diagnosis, timely treatment and culturally sensitive care. Interventions, which address the unique needs of the diverse population of Muslim women may improve outcomes for survivorship. Survivorship plans need to address all the variables, including religious factors and the role of family and community, in providing ongoing follow up care to women who lack transportation, have a strong sense of responsibility for family and not being a burden and for whom breast cancer survivorship is still a distant goal or fatalistic idea.

References

Agurs-Collings, T., Dunn, B. K., Browne, D., Johnson, K. A., & Lubet, R. (2010). Epidemiology of health disparities in relation to the biology of estrogen-receptor-negative breast cancer. *Seminars in Oncology, 37*, 384–401.

American Cancer Society (2015). *Survivorship care plans*. American Cancer Society Information Center, Atlanta, GA.

Bushfield, S., & Fitzpatrick, T. (2010). Therapeutic Interventions with Immigrant Muslim Families in the United States. *Journal of Religion & Spirituality in Social Work, 29*(2), 165–179.

Cedolini, C. (2014). Type of breast cancer diagnosis, screening, and survival. *Clinical Breast Cancer, 14*(4), 235–240.

Centers for Disease Control (CDC) and Prevention, Cancer Screening (2012). *Morbidity and Mortality Report, 61*(3), 41–45.

Centers for Disease Control and Prevention (CDC), Cancer screening United States (2015). U.S. Department of Human Services Centers for Disease Control and Prevention and National Cancer Institute: Atlanta.

Coldman, A. J., & Phillips, N. (2014). Breast cancer survival and prognosis by screening history. *British Journal of Cancer, 110*(3), 556–559.

Dasgupta, P., Baade, P., Aitken, J., Turrell, G. (2012). Multilevel determinants of breast cancer survival: association with geographic remoteness and area-level socioeconomic disadvantage. *Breast Cancer Research and Treatment, 132*(2), 701–710.

DeSantis, C., et al. (2011). Breast cancer statistics. *Cancer Journal 61*(6), 409–418.

Fitzpatrick, T. R., Edgar, L., & Holcroft, C. (2012). Assessing the relationship between physical fitness activities, cognitive health and quality of life among older breast cancer survivors. *Journal of Psychosocial Oncology, 30*, 556–572.

Garofalo, J. P., Choppola, S., Hamann, H., Gjerde, J., (2009). Uncertainty during the transition from cancer patient to survivor. *Cancer Nursing, 32*(4), E8–E14.

Grabler, P., Dupuy, D., Raj, J., Bernstein, S., & Ansell, D. (2012). Regular screening mammography before the diagnosis of breast cancer reduces black/white breast cancer differences and modifies negative prognostic factors. *Breast Cancer Research and Treatment, 135*, 549–553.

Guadalupe, K & Lum, D. (2005). *Multidimensional Contextual Practice.* Belmont, CA: Brooks Cole.

Haddad, Y. (2006). *Muslim women in America: The challenge of Islamic identity today.* Oxford, UK: Oxford University Press.

Harper-Dorton, K & Lantz, J. (2007). *Cross-cultural practice with diverse populations* (2nd ed.) Chicago, Il: Lyceum Books.

Hasnain, M., Menon, U., Ferrans, C. E., & Szalacha, L. (2014). Breast cancer screening practices among first generation immigrant muslim women. *Journal of Women's Health, 23*(7), 602–612.

Hebdon, M., Foli, K., & McComb, S. (2015). Survivor in the cancer context. *Journal of Advanced Nursing, 71*(8), 1774–1786.

Helgeson, V. (2011). Survivor centrality among breast cancer survivors: implications for well being. *Psychooncology, 20*(5), 517–524.

Hodge, D. R. (2005). Social work and the house of Islam: Orienting practitioners to the beliefs and values of Muslims in the United States. *Social Work, 50*(2), 162–173.

Hodge, D. R., & Bushfield, S. Y. (2006). Developing spiritual competence in practice. *Journal of Ethnic and Cultural Diversity in Social Work, 15*(3/4), 101–127.

Jack, R. H., Davies, E. A., & Moller, H. (2009). Breast cancer incidence, stage, treatment and survival in ethnic groups in South East England. *British Journal of Cancer,* 100(3), 545–550.

Jones, B. A., Dailey, A., & Calvocoressi, L. (2005). Inadequate follow-up of abnormal screening mammograms: Findings from the race differences in screening mammography process study. *Cancer Causes and Control, 16*, 809–821.

Koenig, H. G., & Bussing, A. (2010). The Duke University Religion Index (DUREL): A five-item measure for use in epidemiological studies. *Religions, 1*, 78–85.

Koenig, H. G., King, D.E., & Carson, V.B., (2011). *Handbook of Religion and Health*, 2nd ed. New York, NY: Oxford University Press.

Kohler, B. A., et al. (2015). Annual report to the nation on the status of cancer 1975–2011. *Journal of the National Cancer Institute,* 107(6), djv048.

Lum, D. (2003). *Culturally competent practice* (2nd ed.). Belmont, CA: Thomson Brooks/Cole.

Lund, M. J., Brawley, O. P., Ward, K. C., Young, J. L., Gabram, S. S., & Eley, J. W. (2008). Parity and disparity in first course treatment of invasive breast cancer. *Breast Cancer Research and Treatment, 109*, 545–557.

Matin, M., & LeBaron, S. (2004). Attitudes toward cervical cancer screening among Muslim women: A pilot study. *Women and Health, 39*(3), 63–77.

Maxwell, T., & Aldredge-Clanton, J. (1994). Survivor guilt in cancer patients: A pastoral perspective. *Journal of Pastoral Care, 48*(1), 25–31.

Miller, W. R., & Thoresen, C. E. (2003). Spirituality, religion, and health: An emerging research field. *American Psychologist, 58*(1), 24–35.

Mollica, M., & Nemeth, L. (2015). Transition from patient to survivor in African American breast cancer survivors. *Cancer Nursing, 38*(1), 16–22.

Morioka-Douglas, N., Sacks, T., & Yeo, G. (2004). Issues in caring for Afghan American elders: insights from literature and a focus group. *Journal of Cross Cultural Gerontology,*, 19(1), 27–40.

Morris, B., Leporte, S., Wilson, B., Lieberman, M., Dunn, J., & Chambers, S. (2014). *Journal of Cancer Survivorship, 8*(3), 427–436.

Natarajan, L., et al. (2009). Time-varying effects of prognostic factors associated with disease-free survival in breast cancer. *Journal of Epidmiology, 169*, 1463–1470.

National Cancer Institute (2014). *Cancer screening overview for health professionals.* National Institute of Health, Bethesda, MD.

Naus, M., Ishler, M., Parrott, C., & Kovacs, S. (2009). Cancer survivor adaptation. *Journal of Clinical Psychology, 65*(12), 1350–1359.

Olivetto, I., Gomi, A., & Bancej, C. (2002). Influence of delay to diagnosis on prognosic indicators of screen-detected breast carcinoma. *Cancer, 94*, 2143–2150.

Padela, A. I., & Curlin, F. A. (2012). Religious values and healthcare accommodations: Voices from the American Muslim community. *Journal of General Internal Medicine, 27*(6), 709–715.

Padela, A. I., & Curlin, F. A. (2013). Religion and disparities: Considering the influences of Islam on the health of American Muslims. *Journal of Religion and Health, 52*(4), 1333–1345.

Padela, A., Murrar, S., Adviento, B., Liao, C., Hosseinian, Z, Peek ,M., & Curlin, F. (2015). Associations between religion-related factors and breast cancer screening among American Muslims. *Immigrant Minority Health,* 17: 660–669.

Park, C., Zlateva, I., & Blank, T. (2009). Self identity after cancer: "survivor", "victim", "patient", and "person with cancer". *Journal of General Internal Medicine, 24*(Supp 2), S430–S435.

Peek, M. E., & Han, J. H. (2004). Disparities in screening mammography: Current status, interventions and implications. *Journal of General Internal Medicine, 19*(2), 184–194.

Rashidi, A., & Rajaram, S. (2000). Middle Eastern Asian Islamic women and breast self-examination. *Cancer Nursing, 23*(1), 64–70.

Rosedale, M. (2009). Survivor loneliness of women following breast cancer. *Oncology Nursing Forum, 36*(2), 175–183.

Salman, K. F. (2012). Health beliefs and practices related to cancer screening among Arab Muslim women in an urban community. *Health Care for Women International, 33*(1), 45–74.

Shirazi, M., Shirazi, A., & Bloom, J. (2013). Developing a culturally competent faith-based framework to promote breast cancer screening among Afghan immigrant women. *Journal of Religion and Health, 54*, 153–159.

Taplin, S. H., Yabrokk, K. R., & Zapka, J. A. (2012). A multilevel research perspective on cancer care delivery: The example of follow-up to an abnormal mammogram. *Cancer Epidemiological Biomarkers, 21*(1), 1–7.

Zeilani, R. & Seymour, J. E. (2012). Muslim women's narratives about bodily change and care during critical illness: A qualitative study. *Journal of Nursing Scholarship, 44* (1), 99–107.

Chapter 6
Exploring the Artist's Book: How Art Therapy Can Benefit the Quality of Life of Young Adult Breast Cancer Survivors

Katherine Laux

Introduction

This research project explores how six young women with a diagnosis of breast cancer approached the multi-faceted artist's fold book within an art therapy group. An art-based support group for young women living with various stages of breast cancer is a rare opportunity to understand the impact of cancer specific to young women. The Canadian Cancer Society (2010) notes that while the percentage of young people living with cancer is small in comparison to older populations, the impact on the patient and their loved ones and society is huge: Cancer in the young is unexpected and poses great difficulty and interruption in their life. Social relationships, educational pursuits, and careers may be sidetracked as a cancer diagnosis has a major impact on early and young adult responsibilities. Furthermore, the inability to have children, or challenges in raising children, pose a unique loss not felt by older women.

With the pilot project of Laux (2009) as a starting point, this present study utilized a one-time 8-week group to explore the artist's fold book with six young women aged 24–49 years old. Half the women were diagnosed with stage 3, and at the close of the study, at least two had had recent recurrences of stage 4 breast cancer. One recently died in early 2015.

Demographics

The Canadian Cancer Society (2009) reports that 2075 young adults between the ages of 15 and 29 years are diagnosed with cancer each year. For Canadian women

K. Laux (✉)
Cedars CanSupport, 1001 Decarie Blvd., Montreal, QC H4A 3J1, Canada
e-mail: artcanheal@gmail.com

T.R. Fitzpatrick (ed.), *Treating Vulnerable Populations of Cancer Survivors: A Biopsychosocial Approach*, DOI 10.1007/978-3-319-32364-0_6

under the age of 40, there will be an estimated 950 new breast cancer cases this year while in the 40–49 year age group, there will be 3500 new cases according to the Canadian Breast Cancer Foundation (2010).

According to the Canadian Breast Cancer Foundation (2014), close to 20 % of all women newly diagnosed with breast cancer are under 50 years old. A US-based study (Anders et al. 2009), found that approximately one third of all breast cancers are diagnosed in women who are pre-menopausal. Because these women are not regularly screened due to their age, their cancer tends to be more advanced and aggressive by the time of diagnosis. In particular, stage 4 cancer, often referred to as metastatic cancer or advanced cancer, is more prevalent in young women. Anders et al. (2009) report that there is a tendency for breast cancer in young women to be more aggressive, with a poorer prognosis than in post-menopausal women. Medically, younger women represent a "unique biologic entity" with specific concerns such as psychosocial impacts, pregnancy, infertility, bone health, and inherited genetic syndromes which must be addressed in treatment plans (surgical, adjuvant, and psychosocial). These authors stress the need for clinical trials specific to young adults to facilitate better outcomes.

Literature Review

Literature from a variety of disciplines indicates that a diagnosis of breast cancer is a life-altering event, which can have a negative impact on psychological well-being and create psychosocial challenges (Davis 2004; Knobf 2007; Turner et al. 2005). As integrative cancer care expands as awareness increases around the need for whole-patient care, patients' use of complementary and alternative medicine (CAM) as an adjunct to surgery, chemotherapy, hormonal treatments, and radiotherapy is continuing to grow, especially among younger adults and breast cancer patients (Boon et al. 2007; Bennett et al. 2009). Such therapies include practices like yoga, reiki, and meditation; support groups based in creative and expressive arts therapies; and individual services specifically designed to address the needs of cancer patients.

The present research project focuses on the use of group art therapy for young women patients diagnosed with breast cancer. The goals of this study included an exploration of possible benefits, such as alleviating or addressing issues of depression, anxiety, hopelessness, fatigue, and other emotional and physical disturbances resulting from cancer and its treatment effects. Few studies exist investigating the specific benefits of art therapy among young women with breast cancer. Researchers (Ohlen and Rohm 2006) have also noted that patient support groups have traditionally revolved around the needs of older women. Support groups for younger women with breast cancer and their families should be further developed to address age-specific concerns which may arise in connection with major impacts in intimate relationships, infertility, childrearing and motherhood, disruptions in college education, and employment.

Biopsychosocial Impacts of a Breast Cancer Diagnosis for Young Women Depression

According to Wong-Kim and Bloom (2005), younger women under the age of 50 years have greater difficulty coping with a breast cancer diagnosis in comparison to older women, and experience more distress, depression, and a decreased quality of life. These authors note that younger women have greater responsibilities, trying to maintain careers and relationships as well as balancing family life (especially for young mothers), and therefore there are more demands on their time than with older women. They also found that younger women rarely deal with thoughts of their own mortality as older women do. Using a *biopsychosocial* model, Wong-Kim and Bloom conclude that young women who have high levels of pain, low levels of self-esteem, and a lack of perceived emotional support had the greatest risk of depression. These authors recommend that interventions be available for at-risk young women to prevent depressive symptoms from escalating into major depression, which could significantly impact women's quality of life or even end in suicide. Shaha and Bauer-Wu (2009) observe that young women breast cancer survivors contemplate death and dying, and how their illness will affect family and partners as well as their own careers. In their qualitative study using an expressive writing intervention, the following themes were derived: being remembered, landscape of emotions and perspectives, and the omnipresence of life's finitude (Shaha and Bauer-Wu 2009).

Fertility and Childrearing

Cancer treatments can lead to infertility plus other reproductive issues specific to young women. In Connell et al.'s (2006) longitudinal constructionist-based qualitative study of young women under the age of 41, interviews were used to assess thoughts and perceptions of infertility, and whether fertility was regained or not over a period of 12–18 months. For women who regained fertility, pregnancy, and breastfeeding caused fear and anxiety over recurrence and the inability to detect cancer in engorged breasts, as well as fears of bringing up children as a parent with a life-threatening illness. The authors stress the need for young women to have access to relevant information about reproductive issues following a breast cancer diagnosis, and access to counselling services when they experience fear and anxiety surrounding these issues.

For young women who have young children at time of diagnosis, the impact on the women and their families can be staggering. In Ohlen and Rohm's (2006) qualitative study of young women with dependent children, the women shared stories of desolation at having no room for their changing existence. These women felt that their needs were neglected by health practitioners, and also often experienced dissociation from spouses and partners who were unable to adapt to their changing situation. In addition, there were feelings of dissociation related to their experience as an ill or "abnormal" mother, and a sense of disconnection from their bodies and selves. Ohlen and Rohm found that providing a support network exclusively for mothers of dependent children allowed women and their families to move from stories of desolation to stories of consolation. This allows for life transformation while establishing a place to talk about difficult topics such as death and dying, divorce and separation, and the inability to fulfil the role of mother and partner. These authors advocate providing support to the entire family in order to acknowledge and adapt to the changing existence of all family members, especially when partners and other family members are holding onto a previous existence which now cannot be maintained.

Complementary and Alternative Medicine (CAM)

Complementary and alternative medicine (CAM) encompasses a wide array of treatment modalities, which can include body-based work (massage, acupuncture, reiki, yoga, and chiropractic), herbs and diet, creative arts therapies, and support groups. Patients with cancer have been seeking therapies complementary to the use of traditional medicine for years to aid their healing process and improve overall total health (Cassileth and Deng 2004; Richardson et al. 2000). Since the use of CAM is becoming more widespread, physicians are informing themselves in order to offer such opportunities to their patients (Ben-Arye et al. 2008). Furthermore, many recent studies also indicate that breast cancer patients with overall increased quality of life demonstrate longer survival rates (Gupta et al. 2007). Such data is drawing attention to CAM, and endeavours to scientifically investigate the true impact and potential of such therapies is increasing. There is a strong need to investigate the benefits of art therapy for patients living with cancer, especially among young adults.

In *Complementary Therapies: A Guide for People with Cancer* (2014), the Canadian Cancer Society makes a distinction between complementary and alternative medicine. They report that complementary treatments work in conjunction with conventional treatments, whereas alternative treatments are used to replace conventional treatments. While art therapy can be considered a form of complementary treatment, it can also be considered an integral part of cancer care, playing a key role in integrative medicine at many hospitals and cancer care centres that offer art therapy as part of a team of practitioners offering both conventional and complementary treatments and therapies. According to Boon et al. (2007), the use of CAM, including self-medication and working with CAM practitioners, increased over the period from 1998 to 2005. They found that more than 80 % of women with breast cancer were using CAM in 2005 (versus 67 % in 1998) and that these modalities should not be considered alternative treatments any longer due to their prevalence. Boon et al. note that the increased use of CAM calls for increased research to ensure that these treatments are safe and beneficial for breast cancer patients. They write that patients and doctors need to be well-versed of the different modalities available, and make sure the patients are well informed and are comfortable sharing with their doctors their use of CAM.

Bennett et al. (2009) have found that cancer survivors who accessed cancer information were close to six times more likely to use CAM than patients who did not seek out cancer information. They found that younger persons (60 years or younger) accessed more information than older populations and that searching for information online via the internet was more common among younger cancer survivors.

Art Therapy and Art-as-Therapy (Art-Making)

A number of authors have noted the benefits of art-making in a supportive environment for women with breast cancer (Collie et al. 2006; Predeger 1996; Serlin et al. 2000). The literature reveals a lack of patient-centred knowledge on how these women can benefit from visual artistic expression (Collie et al. 2006). The present study has provided an opportunity for young women with breast cancer to share, in their own voices, their experiences making art together. It provides a voice for the participants and thus informs the research from their perspective. It is hoped that this study will add support for the use of art therapy as a means of addressing quality-of-life issues among young women patients with breast cancer. The widespread applicability of our research to other oncology programs may propel the development of art therapy programs specific to young women (or young adults) and other support-based groups to be routinely offered to our AYA patients and their loved ones.

Art Therapy in Oncology

Art therapy includes the use of art-making such as painting, photography, and sculpting and is integrated with psychotherapeutic techniques to promote awareness and creative expression of sentiments (Malchiodi 1999). Art therapy can be used in both individual and group settings in a hospital, home, or community cancer care setting. In cancer care, art therapy can be used with both in- and outpatients, as well as with their caregivers and family members; it can be used just after a cancer diagnosis, during chemo treatments and post-treatment, and during the palliative phase. Malchiodi defines medical art therapy as a mind–body intervention, which supports the "power of the mind to influence the body in ways which encourage and stimulate health and well-being (p. 17)". According to Bocking (2005), her chief role as an art therapist at a London hospital with in- and outpatients being treated for cancer is to "hold a safe space" to explore life and death issues and explore the uncertainty and the unknowingness of a cancer diagnosis.

Art Therapy and Meaning-Making

Collie et al. (2006) also write that breast cancer can cause a broad range of psychosocial difficulties such as a change in lifestyle, interpersonal relationship strains, social isolation, and existential emergencies, and can impact a woman's ability to find and create meaning. Breast cancer, according to Collie et al., can diminish a woman's ability to create meaning and to create life stories that are purposeful. A number of researchers investigating the benefits of art-making and art therapy for women with breast cancer have focused on a process known as "meaning-making" (Bell 2006; Collie et al. 2006; Collie and Long 2005; Laux 2009; Predeger 1996; Taylor 2000).

Collie and Long (2005) define meaning-making as "an ongoing process of storying to create and maintain a coherent life story that casts the self as valuable, unique and permanent" (p. 762). Also, there is strong evidence that the ability to successfully reconstruct a self and world view with purpose and order in life can lead to improved adjustment and quality of life in patients with cancer (Bower et al. 2005; Carpenter 1999; Kissane et al. 2007; Lee 2008; Taylor 2000). Opportunities such as support groups or individual sessions to encourage emotional and cognitive processing are essential to the meaning-making process to aid in transforming distress into psychological growth (Breitbart et al. 2010; Lee et al. 2006).

In Laux's (2009) earlier study of older women diagnosed with breast cancer, the data included artwork, discussions arising within group sessions, case notes, and follow-up narrative-based interviews. Qualitative data analysis of the interviews resulted in four major themes: *Breaking Down the Isolation*; *Emotional Awakenings*; *Structure and Freedom to Explore*; and *Realizing Capabilities.* Laux (2009) described a unique art-therapeutic intervention to aid in meaning-making and to address the psychosocial and emotional disruptions that may occur following a recent breast cancer diagnosis. Although some initial research has been done in this domain, there is much room for further inquiry, especially by incorporating the authentic voices of younger adult participants on how they can benefit from art-making and the exhibition of artworks. How could exhibits or public displays of artworks benefit young women living with cancer? How might they benefit the viewer and their perceptions of young women living with cancer? Overall, the interesting and promising field of art therapy requires more scientifically structured assessments, through mixed methods inquiries and utilizing innovative qualitative analysis, to reveal its true potential for the health and well-being of young oncology patients.

Methodology

Study Design: This pilot study began with a qualitative and quantitative component. Over time, however, it became clear through feedback from the participants that the quantitative questionnaires would not be useful in answering our research queries.

Some participants did not answer them correctly, and some not at all. The challenges of administering questionnaires were also noted in a concurrent study in art therapy in oncology at the MUHC and are currently being explored (Lee et al. 2015). In the end, the qualitative measure was used in evaluating an intervention group of six young women receiving art therapy over the course of 8 weeks, with individual narrative-based interviews following post-group. Although the group was originally planned for 6 weeks, it became necessary to extend the group to accommodate both missed sessions and give more time to complete the projects. The impacts of the chemotherapy and radiation treatments were strongly felt, and more time and flexibility were needed in the group space.

Setting

Art therapy sessions took place in the art room at a Cancer Wellness Centre in Montreal, Quebec, Canada. The conference room had four tables and ample chairs to accommodate up to eight art-making participants. A locked cabinet in the adjoining library safely contained the participant artworks for the duration of the study. All artwork belonged to the artists and was returned to them post-group. In November and December 2011, the art room was booked once a week for two to three hours, for a period of eight weeks.

Subjects/Patients and Recruitment

Initially, 12 young female patients were recruited from the Cancer Wellness Centre for this pilot study to ensure a final intervention group with eight women patients. Flyers describing the study were available at the reception desk of the centre and distributed to members of the treating team at the local affiliated hospital. With the guidance and discretion of staff and volunteers at the Wellness Centre and the hospital, information about this study was shared with young women recently diagnosed with breast cancer. Interested patients were asked if they agreed to be contacted by the art therapist by either phone or by email. The art therapist followed up with all interested patients, briefed them on the study, and answered any questions. Additional time was added at the beginning of the first group session and at the last session to go over the consent form and fill out the assessments, with ample time for any questions/concerns to be addressed. Nine women signed up for the group but after the group started, only six women were able to attend regularly. Consent forms were administered with the approval of the hospital Institutional Review Board (IRB). The forms were then locked a safe place in the research office at the Wellness Centre.

Inclusion Criteria

1. Women 18–45 years
2. Stage I to III breast cancer
3. Minimum of 6 weeks Post Operative status
4. English and/or French speakers

The literature covers a range of ages for the population encompassing the term *young adults*, and Cancer Care Ontario (2006) notes that there is no standard definition for young adults. Some articles use the terminology adolescent and young adult (AYA) which can include the ages 15–29, while others use the term young adult to include ages 19–44, others use under 50 or even under 60 years of age. One study using focus groups and interviewing, Dunn and Steginga (2002) found that women with breast cancer defined as "young" any woman of childbearing age, whether childless or with young (primary-school or younger) children, who has not yet reached menopause. For the purpose of this study, we focused on ages 18–45 years, with some flexibility to include women who may choose to have children (biologically or not) at an older age (mid to late forties).

Intervention

The art therapy sessions were 2–3 h in duration, with 1 session/week for eight continuous weeks. The focus of the group was to explore the expressive capabilities of art-making in a highly structured environment as outlined by Luzzatto and Gabriel (2000) and successfully implemented and explored in an earlier study (Laux 2009). Each session began with a brief check-in to assess how participants were feeling as they entered the safe therapeutic space. Each session focused on a theme chosen by the group that reflected the needs of women who were in treatment for breast cancer, which included exploring and releasing difficult emotions (Collie et al. 2006); addressing existential crises (Landmark and Wahl 2002); exploring the ever-changing connection between body and mind (Bell 2006; Lemieux et al. 2008; Serlin et al. 2000); and finding one's inner strength and meaning-making capabilities as one journeys through the cancer experience (Collie et al. 2006; Predeger 1996).

A guided visualization followed the check-in to help each participant relax and focus her mind, and to introduce the art-based intervention. Art-making followed for about an hour. A broad range of art media were laid out at each session, including high quality papers of various textures in a range of dimensions, oil/chalk pastels, pencils, tempera/acrylic paints, brushes, tissue papers, boxes, mirror tiles, beads, glitter, fabric/yarns, photo collage materials, glue, clay, wire, and an assortment of natural materials (such as leaves, twigs, sand, shells, and seeds). After art-making, artwork was presented for viewing, and a group share followed to give space for exploring their creative process and emotions/thoughts that came up. At the close of the session, a short checkout was used to assess how participants were feeling as they left the session, and to make sure that everyone was emotionally grounded.

During the reflection/discussion part of the art therapy session, the following questions/suggestions were posed each week: *Please share with the group what it is that you are depicting? What was it like to do this exercise? Did any thoughts or emotions come up when you were making art today? Please share if you feel comfortable. If you would like more feedback, you can invite others to share their thoughts on your artwork.* While the session discussions were semi-structured in nature, with pre-selected questions guiding the inquiry, the art therapist remained open to the ebb and flow of each session and the unique experience of each woman.

Demographic Information

Demographic data and disease characteristics are presented in Table 1 (see Appendix). The average age of the women was 38.8 years old with a range of 24 to 49 years. Initially, we proposed to use both qualitative and quantitative tools in order to evaluate the impact of the intervention. In order to assess the main outcome variable of Quality of Life (QOL), we used measures for pre- and post-testing to compare the difference between the two time periods and assess whether there had been positive changes in QOL at the post-test. The women were generally not pleased to fill out the quantitative questionnaires. Several did not fill out or complete the pre- and post-measures. A few would pick a range of values for their answers. They found that numbers could not evaluate how they were feeling or doing or their experiences or beliefs. They felt more comfortable sharing their thoughts during the session and in post-group interviews and hand-written responses. Therefore, this data was not used in the analyses.

Objective 1: To investigate qualitatively how group art therapy using the artist's fold book can improve the QOL of young women with breast cancer, including the challenges of finding and creating meaning following a breast cancer.

Post-group interview questions for qualitative analysis	
1	Please share with me your experience of making art in the group. What was it like?
2	Was there a particular artwork or theme that you found special or more meaningful? If so, can you tell me more about it?
3	Did art-making or art therapy assist you as you journeyed through your cancer diagnosis and treatment (or post-treatment)? If so, please elaborate
4	How did you find working with the book or doll form, or any of the different media (painting, collage, sculpture…)?
5	Is there anything else you would like to share?
6	Do you have suggestions for future art-based support groups for young women living with breast cancer?
7	Would you be interested in exhibiting any of your artworks anonymously? If yes, would you prefer to create artworks for the exhibit in a separate open studio session, or would you prefer to use an artwork from this 8-week group?

Table 1 Demographic information for sample of young women survivors

	Demographic information for sample of young women survivors (N = 6)			
		n	Mean	Range
Age			38.8 years	24–49 years
	20s	1		
	30s	1		
	40s	4		
Marital/Relationship status	Has partner	1		
	No partner	5		
Children	Yes	2		
	No	4		
Date of diagnosis	December 2010	2		
	January–June 2011	3		
	August 2011	1		
Stage			2.5	1–3
	1	1		
	2/3	2		
	3	3		
Post-study—two of the women became stage 4 and one died in 2015 due to her illness				
Breast surgery type	Lumpectomy	1		
	Mastectomy	5		
Treatments: chemo, radiation, hormonal	Chemo and radiation	6		
	Hormonal	3		

Qualitative Inquiry: Description

With the informed consent of participants, the art therapist/researcher took photographs of artwork, as well as case notes written from observations during art-making and any discussions that took place during the group. In addition, narrative-based one-on-one interviews by the researcher took place following the group sessions and, with permission granted, the interviews were recorded. All artworks created during the group remained the intellectual property of each participant and were returned at the end of the interviews. A larger group exhibit open to all women living with breast cancer took place in October 2013 through Cedars CanSupport, Montreal, QC. All the artists were invited to participate and exhibit their artwork anonymously; two of those six artists ultimately agreed to show their art, while using a pseudonym. However, this was not part of the present study.

Narrative Inquiry

A narrative inquiry guided this study, both for the art therapy group discussions and for the post-group interviews. Polkinghorne (1988) writes that to best understand human beings, the human sciences have to realize the primacy of narrative in the lives of people, in their experiences and existence. Polkinghorne states that narrative inquiry provides the tools to understand people's storied lives. Josselson and Lieblich (2003) write that the goal in narrative is to "create interpreted description of the rich and multi-layered meanings of historical and personal events… the search is for truths unique in their particularity" (p. 259), so as to create and expand on concepts, and to inform others. In narrative inquiry, the researcher has to remain open to discovery by involving themselves in a process of capturing the lived experiences of others, and their meaning-making. Neuman (2006) describes the narrative inquiry as one that captures peoples' ordinary lives; the researcher is self-reflective and gets involved in the plot as a co-participant in the study. Marshall and Rossman (2006) refer to the openness and trust involved between the researcher and participant in narrative inquiry. Marshall and Rossman write that the relationship between researcher and participant is mutually collaborative and takes significant time to develop so as to fully understand the participant's experiences.

Qualitative Analysis

Qualitative analysis of the narrative-based interviews followed, using Neuman's (2006) step-by-step approach to coding data to seek out and understand the major themes and types of meaning-making that the participants address in their art-making, and in their narratives about their journey with cancer as a whole. The process began with open coding of each line or chunk of text (transcribed interviews, open-ended questions, artwork, notes) to help bring potential themes to the surface from a range of data. We then moved to axial coding, where potential connections and links are explored and themes are further refined. The process ends with selective coding, where select cases in the data illuminate the codes/themes and validate the coding-based qualitative analysis.

Lincoln and Guba (1985) proposed four criteria (credibility, transferability, dependability, and confirmability) for judging the soundness of qualitative research as alternatives to the more traditional quantitatively oriented criteria of validity and reliability. Validity and reliability were addressed by use of prolonged engagement with the research participants, triangulation of data sources, member checks (having participants review and approve transcribed discussions and derived themes), peer debriefing, and use of thick description and contextual details, and the use of a reflexive journal to track personal biases and expectations.

Results/Discussion

The goal of this study was to investigate how art therapy focusing on the artist's book format can facilitate expression and meaning-making and improve quality of life among young women breast cancer survivors. The qualitative data analysis described here provided answers to this question by bringing into focus certain recurring themes in the participants' experience of the group and their creative process. After analyzing the interviews in light of the sessions, case notes, and artwork, the analysis of the narrative-based interviews using Neuman's (2006) method yielded four major themes and some sub-themes: (1) *Unspeakable losses* and *challenging the face of cancer*; (2) *Two selves*; (3) *On her own terms*, and (4) *Connections.*

The following presents the themes as they are discussed with selected quotations from the individual interviews or in reflection of the artwork or shared discussions. A subsidiary research question is also discussed throughout, e.g.: What symbols predominate in the artworks of young women with breast cancer?

Unspeakable Losses and Challenging Stereotypes

In the theme of unspeakable losses faced by the young women, the following quotes from the interviews address the point—"*It's not nothing*" [i.e. what I'm going through is more significant than some might think] *and* '*I got a timeline*' [i.e. I have to plan my life around the fact of my imminent mortality]. Also relevant here is a related theme of 'challenging the face of cancer'. When hearing, through voice and image, the stories that the young women shared about their experiences being diagnosed, and all the impacts and losses they experienced, one cannot help but see the overwhelming number of symbols relating to their pain and loss. Teardrops, wounds, blood drops, internal body workings and venous imagery, fear, hair loss, and jagged lines predominated. The painful inner workings and effects of the cancer are brought to the surface. The invisible becomes visible. Through these symbols and discussion with the young women, they challenge the face of cancer.

For young women undergoing chemo, early onset of menopause and infertility are common. One woman spoke of being pushed into menopause artificially, and of a lack of opportunity to progress or age naturally. This hurt deeply. The teardrop, blood drop, or chemo drop were featured in several of her artworks (*Example 1—See Artwork Appendix*). The same woman used the teardrop form when referring to her chemo treatments. She spoke about the physiological and emotional impacts by saying "*All the inside of me was a whole universe of things going on and it felt that if I pushed myself, I would ignite a big bang so it seemed best to not push myself and just to let things seep*". She referred to feeling poisoned and '*freaked out*'. She continued by saying '*I was being hit from behind almost ... with that deep sense, that deep mortality trip that comes. That really deep, like incredibly open sense of possibility that I could not wake up tomorrow, and being the single parent and not having all my affairs in order*".

Infertility and motherhood were common themes in the group. Two of the women were single mothers struggling to raise children alone while battling their illness. The others tried to grapple with the inability to have children following their treatments (infertility or early menopause). One woman underwent procedures to conserve her eggs before treatment. It proved unsuccessful and highly unlikely that her eggs would survive for future pregnancies. '*It's not nothing*' to go through any of this, she said. She was able to explore this loss through a body-based book exercise. She said it was '*very important to speak of the unspeakable*'. She spoke about her purple-paper-covered three page book as containing herself on the exterior, with the outside brown layer reflecting how she was actually feeling, and a raw interior depicting her scars and her loss following surgery and chemo treatments. The interior page was a pink sheet representing cancer. She said the book allowed for layers of complexity—internal, external, and real. She was surprised to find out how much could be processed through the symbolic as opposed to verbal means alone. In the same body-based book, she also explored how breast cancer alters the body, how it can alter significantly, and that as long as you are alive this is a loss even if you decide to do reconstruction. She spoke of the need to grieve this loss, and that she is still grieving. For her, the book validated the loss. She also depicted an 'x' to mark the spot—period gone, menstruation ended. She was put into early menopause. She said multiple times—'*It's not ok.*' (*Example 2—See Artwork Appendix*).

Another woman had more advanced cancer, and after a lengthy process to obtain a proper diagnosis, she moved from her own province to Montreal to get proper treatment. Given the advanced state of her cancer, she was discouraged from considering any fertility preservation. Emphasis was placed on starting treatments as soon as possible to save her life. Having children was not an option. The loss was profound. Loss was a common theme, including the loss of an intact body.

In addition to the impacts of losing fertility or losing a breast, the loss of hair was another profound loss. One found the loss of her hair a threat to her femininity, and she went to great extents to hide the loss of her hair through wigs and hats. '*Chemo has just taken the very thing that made me feel like a woman*'. In her drawings made at home, chemo was depicted as arrows trying to kill the once vibrant woman she had been. Her hair was a huge part of her pride and identity. During her treatments, she kept her illness to herself, even with close friends. One friend, wanting to start a more serious intimate relationship with her, decided not to pursue relations beyond friendship after hearing of her diagnosis. For women in relationships or wanting to find intimate relationships, it is very challenging for both to work through all the unknowns and impacts of the illness (loss of a breast, infertility, treatment side effects, and for those living with advanced cancer, treatments for life).

The impact of building camaraderie between the women was felt. Midway through the group, this same woman took her wig off; this was the first time she had ever revealed her baldness to anyone outside of a hospitalization for infection. Wearing the wig did afford this young woman with a chance to feel more normal.

She could drink coffee with her neighbours and feel part of the community without disclosing her illness. She desperately wanted to feel normal. She coped through disguise. However, the group space afforded her the opportunity to share the unspeakable loss of her hair. Her struggles with hair loss can be seen in her doll, which had two faces and two sets of hair, or hair and baldness. One face is sad, with a wrap covering her head masking her baldness. On the other side is her happy face with long braided hair (*Example 3—See Artwork Appendix*).

Another challenge she carried was feeling that there was a timeline for her life. '*I got a timeline. There's two sides. It might come up, it might not. 10 years. 20. 30? How do you plan your life when you have to build it around a timeline?*' This was a huge disruption in her work life, and with her continued low energy even many months after treatment, she was struggling with her fear of not being independent anymore, especially financially. What would happen if she could not return to work? She was single and had just moved to Canada; she did not want to depend on family and thus become a dependent.

Another young woman also felt a sense of living a timeline. During the 'chaos and order' exploration, group participants were encouraged to identify a current challenge, such as fear, and then its opposite, e.g. contentment. She chose to depict her feelings about her upcoming mastectomy surgery. Her fear related to the idea that how you will do is measured from date of surgery. Her fear about surgery was depicted as a mechanical or frightening clinical experience. The darkness in her artworks depicted the negatives—death, the unknown, and fear of the dark future. The timeline starts with good healthy days, then gets grayer and darker and finally turns black. Red symbolizes the day of surgery.

Still another woman felt time ticking away, earlier than her naturally allotted time, and had an awareness of something being wrong before diagnosis, a certain kind of intuition.

> Time … it has been quite a while since I have been operating on– that I have been living with this underlying sensation that… 'tick tock. tick tock. tick tock'. I was feeling like that for quite a while before I was aware of having cancer. I kept revisiting it, wondering why it was sitting there and writing about it and stuff. There was something sitting there quite a while before

In her first past, present, and future triptych, the moon (the clock) is the clock-like element, the "*tick-tock*". Through simple books, box-based art, and dolls, the women shared the complexity of their pain and loss. The sensation of a limited time came up frequently, as did challenges with relationships and challenges with motherhood and not being able to be a mother.

Two Selves

This theme revolves around dualities, or a quality of being dual, or a circumstance of opposing or contrasting aspects as they relate to the self. In this theme, struggles with identity predominate. The impacts of a cancer diagnosis are huge, especially when they occur early in adulthood. Many of the women begin reprioritizing what is important, and came to a crossroads where they have to make major life choices and changes.

Career Impacts

One of the young women chose the doll form to share two visions of the future by using two separate heads. She felt that she had to choose between two paths—one that would be beneficial for her teenage son, and one that would be beneficial for herself. She felt obligated to continue her studies to provide for the two of them, but she simultaneously felt that this path might not be the best choice for herself. She felt a lot of questioning. How would she be after treatment? What would the next steps be? How would she be able to continue her studies or work with all the lingering side effects including neuropathy and exhaustion? When referring to her needs and the needs of her teenage son, she spoke of being able to '*fold*' their needs together in the past. But now she felt she had to compromise on what her inner world wanted to be most immersed in or invested in, and what she wanted for her son, '*I could bring them together and they can cohabitate, but it has been going more and more and more like this. It seems like I'm on this track where I'm further and further away from these other things that I value more*'. Her doll with two heads, made with blue and red intertwining pipe cleaners, speaks to figuring out two paths. The two heads are reminiscent of not only the blue and red tears of her other works but of veins and arteries. Because the two heads are part of the same body, it seems telling that both paths are part of her—not unlike Frida Kahlo's work, *Two Fridas,* which we spoke about together during the interview.

This woman's pain, especially neuropathy, can be seen in her Chimaera piece. When speaking about her past as both a dancer and involved in physical theatre she said "*I realized from that first spring back from chemo that my legs are such a big deal... there's some really interwoven thing that I associate with having strength in my legs and agility and the feeling of solidity in my legs, and without it there is an additional vulnerability*". The loss of feeling in her legs brought great fear and questioned her abilities as a performer and dancer—"*...because I have a history as a dancer and physical theatre, my physicality and my identity were so intrinsically intertwined that when I first starting having health problems I actually had an identity crisis*". She had to rethink how she would be or could be as she finished treatments and hoped the neuropathy would not be permanent. Would she be able to continue her work as interdisciplinary artist or dance again or return to her studies?

The patient described above was not alone in using multiple heads or creating hybrid animal imagery. Another woman used doll-making to create a three-headed dragon (*Example 4—See Artwork Appendix*). The doll was her favourite exploration and it took her several weeks to make. It became larger than the doll or animal project—it also became integrated into the past, present, and future triptych activity. A three-headed triptych. The present was the larger head in the centre.

Green was central to making this creature. She spoke of her use of greens as not being a conscious choice but green for her was '*like protection, it's like nature. Trees. The woods and that's really where I feel comfortable*'. For all three women who made dolls with multiple heads—they depicted several states of being or paths or aspects of the self (private and personal) that needed to be explored. While the dragon represented both bird and reptile, another artist created a hybrid fish with a mass of feathers for the head. The fish did not know where it was going—in one direction or another. There is a circle of question marks surrounding the fish. She said that she has been thinking of switching professions or at least improving her old profession. She said she felt passionately about scuba diving and would love to see herself as a scuba diving instructor. It is a huge issue for her right now—trying to figure out a career path that is both satisfying and pays well enough.

On Her Own Terms

The women were actively processing new ways of thinking and moving forward. Better ways of coping and building up protections, and a better, stronger emerging self, and transformations are seen in this category. As the young women worked from week to week and reflected on who they were, who they are, and where they will be through the past, present and future triptych and through their self-portraits in animal and doll and box and book forms—they began to integrate who they were becoming. New forms of coping and a stronger and wiser self were emerging. Some are more subtle and some are larger transformations. One of the many ways in which they were becoming better equipped in their coping was building up protections and boundaries.

Building Protection

Identifying protection, or learning to build protections symbolically and literally, was a common theme. Gold, shields and other containing circle forms and concealing boxes and books, semi-precious stones, crosses, halos, dragons, and nature pop up in the imagery of the group as protective forms. One artist built golden halos or pointy crowns or thick unruly hair adorning her figures. She also coloured in mandalas during her chemo treatments and at home. She wrote: "*I recall the golden bubbles/halos on my past, present, future piece as representing a kind of reflective shield of sorts. Not impenetrable at all, but a psychic emitting/projecting/protecting barrier, nonetheless. The dual, sometimes triple, halo layers indicated to me layers or sometimes alternating psychic states or dispositions.*" (*Example 5—See Artwork Appendix*). Gold and other metals and stones (semi-precious and rhinestones) can be found in paintings, sculpture, and jewellery. One participant wrapped a semi-precious stone with wire and hung it on a cord to wear as a protective amulet. She chose a tumbled Tiger's Eye stone which has associated metaphysical properties of balancing yin and yang energy, and is known for its grounding ability as well as its capacity to enhance clarity and soothe (Melody 1995).

Breaking from Tradition

As the women built up their protections in their art as it corresponded to their lives, they shared a lot of their wishes to move forward in a way that put their own interests and livelihood first. One of these ways was to break from tradition and culture. One artist spoke of living differently from tradition or family. She wanted to be accepted without marrying and to live alone while having a boyfriend, to express herself when women were not supposed to speak their minds or be successful at work. She said "*I'm 41, I need to stand up for myself and without the guilt and burdens of tradition*". She spoke of needing to free herself yet acknowledged that this would be a difficult transition. She referred to her experience of having cancer as not just a sickness, but a transformative experience. She linked having cancer to other difficult life transitions and wondered how it could better inform her future. Although she spoke of being a failure in her parents' eyes (unmarried, childless) and blamed for her own cancer diagnosis, she was determined to be her own person. She set out to find her passion, remain independent and financially sound. She had plans of how to make her dreams of being a scuba diving instructor come true.

Another woman gave up her career as an accountant to take care of kids in her children's school. She was a single mom who wanted to be closer to her children's lives but also to find more meaningful work. She found it very rewarding and felt that the kids gave so much back. Another participant in the group worked hard to maintain her independence from family, even though she could not work. It was important to not regress and return to earlier familial experiences of dependence in youth. In many cases, these young women are just coming into who they are as independent adults when they are faced with cancer.

As far as artistic expression of this theme, one woman created a doll which could be endlessly changed. The doll and a range of materials were stored in a box. Pom-poms of different sizes and colours could be interchanged to change the doll's face (*Example 6—See Artwork Appendix*). She did not want to finish her doll as did the woman who created the two-headed doll. Similarly, the dragon doll described earlier had three heads to represent various parts of the self in different times. The need for multiple faces and creatures (chimaeras) may speak to a self that is very much still developing and grappling for a new identity.

Building Boundaries and Healthier Relationships

Some of the young women braved new careers, while others were developing better personal relationships. For one of the young women, coming to the art therapy group itself was not an easy choice, but she was adamant to brave new relationships —both building relationships with other women like herself, to break up her isolation, but also to share more of her experiences with her loved ones. Although her brother was emotionally distant, she began reaching out to her friends around her. At first, she was unable to share her diagnosis and treatments, but over time she found the courage to share her story, and her friends were very supportive. When her brother told family members about her illness against her wishes, she developed ways to keep some distance. She said '*so I don't have to tell them anything?*' It was her choice. She felt she coped better alone, yet acknowledged the benefits of the group and sharing her story when she was ready, on her own terms. Her imagery reflects this need to hide to prepare, especially in the past, present, and future triptych book. She describes a foetus and womb on one of the pages, which could refer to the need to retreat and the healing potential of solitude, but also to this new life of hers and just starting out again as she moved into post-treatment. She spoke of feeling anxious and nervous and scared and seeking comfort in the mother's womb, which contains warmth and protection. As she was able to brave sharing her story and opening up to friends who embraced her, she was surprised to find out how much they wanted to celebrate her finishing treatments with a big "birthday" celebration. Taking place not on her actual birthday, but to mark the end of a very difficult time, the party served to mark her new life post-treatment. They told her '*You've got a new lease on life!*'. She built a family of her own to support her and be with her through the ups and downs of her illness. Her experiences show the importance of meaningful rituals that women can make for themselves, even if they do not come from family, culture, or tradition.

Connections

This theme includes the connections the women made with each other, while also highlighting the benefits of a space just for young women. As most of the women were in active treatment, the make-up of each session was different. The young women connected well from session to session. They opened up and shared their experiences and lent a lot of support to each other. One woman felt less alone with others in a similar age bracket. She found it soothing and relaxing. Even when she could not make many of the sessions, as she was a single mom just returning to work and embroiled in a custody battle with her ex-partner, she made time to work on the projects at home and got her children involved in the art-making too. Connecting young parents was important. One of the single moms in the group was appreciative to connect with another fellow parent. She said it helped to feel less alone because "*I kind of recognized some of her, something about her that I think I recognize from my own journey of parenthood. At least I can sum it up like that. I only met her that once but...*". The impacts of the group could be felt not only through the children of the single parents, but one of the partners of one woman said she always looked radiant after the group and he encouraged her to keep going. She said she felt systematically better after each session and that she was beginning to return to her giddy old self.

Normalizing Connections

Connecting to a non-diseased part of the self was important, as was a need to return to normalcy. One braved coming to art therapy as she needed to share and be seen as she had not shared her experience with anyone but her brother. She said she could finally say '*I'm not abnormal*' and not have shame. The group experiences meant we were all '*in the same shoes*' and not alone in our experiences. She was able to reveal her bald head in both art and in-person and this was very liberating and allowed her to eventually share with her loved ones. The impact of the supportive space with like young people had a huge impact. She hoped she could educate other young women.

Additional Important Findings: How the Women Used Art Therapy to Their Benefit and Suggestions for the Future

While the creative process for some was deep therapeutic work, others in the group found that making art was important because you did not have to think. You could get lost in the process. The therapeutic art space could hold both deep explorations and losing oneself in art or building beauty through art (Luzzatto 2005). One woman felt that art-making could beautify cancer—providing a way to find some good in all that was happening. She created a stunning hand-painted and glitter-full, nature-based box to hold her cancer slides and original diagnosis. It made her feel that things were not all bad. This woman did not like to share verbally, but was very content opening up and relaxing while making art and surrounded by others like herself. Being among young people was extremely important to her, and this was the only therapy she had sought out because there was the option for introspection and less verbal interaction. She recommended that art therapy options be an ongoing option, not just a research opportunity, and that there should be the additional option of art-based supports specific to young adults. She felt invisible as a young adult. She had tried peer-led studios, but felt that a therapeutic art-based support would be better. She also noted that there were many incomplete projects, and suggested that ongoing art-based supports would attend to the pace of each project and provide further explorations. The other women had the same experience—that it was not possible to attend consecutive sessions. They felt an open group space would be more accommodating than a closed group of limited duration as in this study. Others gave feedback that the sessions should be longer, so that there would be time to talk and connect as well as time to make art. They felt that both aspects were very necessary, but that sometimes the sessions would predominate with discussions and sharing. While necessary, this took up some of the art-making time.

Several of the artists appreciated art-making options that could be taken along to treatments. It helped them to brave treatments alone, made the experience more comforting, and helped to pass the time. Mandalas and knitting were popular choices for portable art-making, in part because they are simple and less demanding ways of making art on the go. When referring to her art therapy experience, one of the women wrote: "*It's more appropriate to your state at the time... Actually every time I try to start something at home it just ends up sitting there and I have an aversion to it... which is exactly the opposite of what I expected from my treatment time, ya know?*" The majority of the group found it easier to make art together rather than at home although some found having '*art therapy assignments*' helped them to continue making art at home especially if they were missing in-person sessions and wanted to participate from home.

Among those more interested in deeper work, such as expressing depth of emotions or expressions of the unconscious, one woman in particular found it both surprising and enriching to access her deep thoughts. She preferred the smaller group size and the fact that no one took offence when the patients could not always attend week after week. She felt the smaller group size made it easier to connect, more comfortable to delve into projects quickly and deeply, and to access the unconscious through art. She found it to be a powerful technique and she appreciated the directive approach. She noted that without some sort of direction or structured activity, she would not have gone there. She would have avoided tough subjects. She said '*imposing subjects*' was useful and that the thinking continued at home.

The women identified the projects that were the most helpful to them. All the women identified with the past, present, and future triptych. One wrote that going to the past was important to understanding the '*now*' and where they were headed. She felt that she had a beautiful life, that the future was green (hopeful and rich) and that art-making put herself first—the load was lifted simply by cutting paper (*Example 7—See Artwork Appendix*). Since she was a single mom of two young sons, she appreciated the focus on herself.

Nature, growth, and the colour green came up a lot as sources of solace, beauty and richness. One woman remarked that the body exercise was a good place to start. She created a self-portrait book with her body superimposed onto a tree. She imagined being healed by nature's medicine pulsing through her veins. It helped her to understand her treatments better if she could relate the treatment to mother nature (*Example 8—See Artwork Appendix*). Nature for her was protection and a place of comfort. A nature scene also adorned her box, which '*held*' her cancer. It became a meaningful place, a beautiful space to hold her slides (and thus her experience). She had previously stored her slides in a paper bag in her closet. This project brought her illness out of the closet, so to speak, and the box could now adorn her dresser.

Several of the women spoke of making art at home between sessions or during treatments and for the need to keep making art after the group ended, to create a creative space at home. As one of them said: "*It's actually a survival mechanism for me. I have to anchor myself to things that are meaningful to me*". Four of the six women continued on with art-making on their own or through open studio and art therapy groups at the hospital. All of them were interested in exhibiting their work and sharing their experiences anonymously.

This qualitative research sought to understand how art-making interventions can facilitate the visual expression of young women's experiences such that they can explore their individual and collective meanings related to their needs and well-being. By finding meaning in their experiences through art-making together, and also highlighting it in exhibition, these women found an important way to bear witness to their experience in both a closed group space and in the larger community. They could safely share the invisible. In creating art, young women have the opportunity to give voice in a creative way that leaves a tangible record of their ongoing exploration of meaning. Both the process of creating art and the final product and exhibition opportunity provide therapeutic value. Furthermore, the exhibition provided an awareness opportunity for the public.

Implications and Future Research

An Adolescent and Young Adult (AYA) specific exhibit would be a nice future exploration, as a way to challenge the traditional face of cancer. It is hoped that this research will contribute to the emerging literature in medical art therapy especially the benefits of providing support spaces for specific sub-groups in cancer care such as young women in treatment for breast cancer. This research provides for both patient and public witnessing of women's efforts towards meaning, thus bringing their experiences into public discourse. Incorporating the voices of the participants in this study, in combination with a group exhibit, will contribute towards patient-centred knowledge about how women with breast cancer benefit from visual artistic expression (Collie et al. 2006).

Conclusions

This study was an essential educational experience to build upon for future groups. The women in our study were forthcoming and generous with their suggestions for future art therapy group work. The ideas for improving the future of support groups in cancer care for young adults were gleaned from group discussions and in individual interviews. While it was interesting to focus on one form of art-making to explore the impacts of group art therapy, a range of media is always important. Some of the women appreciated that book-making had specific unique traits, such as complexity of layers, or the ability to open and close (reveal and conceal) or expand and contain. Others were just as open to other media options as well. The impacts of the treatments were strongly felt within the group, and more time and flexibility were needed in the group space. Simplicity in materials and accomplishing the final artwork is essential, as seen in the literature (Luzzatto 2005). Several of the women thought we should have an additional final session to connect all explorations and projects of the 8-week group into one larger book or box to contain all projects. They thought it could be important to create a larger structure that was a sacred safe space for oneself. It could be concealed but easily opened to reveal when needed. More importantly, they expressed a strong need for ongoing creative arts therapy programming for young adults, especially programming that would be specific to those with advanced cancer. Further exploration of challenging subject matter was suggested as well; suggestions included working with challenging family relationships, sexuality, fertility, and dying/death.

Young Adult Art Therapy Programming

Great strides have been made in the realm of cancer care specific to young adult cancer survivors across Canada and especially in Montreal. Examples include the Cancer Fight Club through the Hope & Cope Wellness Centre, and the AYA support programming developed at Cedars CanSupport. In particular, the results of the study described in this chapter have impacted the work at CanSupport, and have informed the AYA cancer care programming offered there which revolves around creative arts therapies approaches. These new groups and programs have relevance for young breast cancer survivors as well. Several years after this study began, an art therapy group was developed specific to young adults living with metastatic or advanced cancer which was co-developed by one of the participants in this study. In conjunction with this group, there is an Art + Play group offering to parents who take part in the group. Loved ones are also welcome to attend. This AYA group remains an open group, so that all those living with advanced cancer have ongoing support. An open group model also provides more flexibility with ongoing sessions, and the ability to work at a pace that works for each individual. Online support services are currently being explored so that programming remains inclusive and accessible to all in need. Hope & Cope has also developed a family-based program en Famille. Both patient and family supports are being developed for younger adults. For therapists running support groups for adults, understanding the unique impacts our AYAs and especially those with breast cancer, will help oncology professionals to be more inclusive and respectful of the range of needs all our patients and their loved ones present.

Acknowledgments This research project could not have been undertaken without the support of my colleagues at Hope & Cope Wellness Centre and Cedars Can Support. I owe a great deal to Dr. Tanya Fitzpatrick for encouraging me to do this study and for all her insight, guidance, feedback, and availability throughout the research process. Lastly, I want to thank the women of this study who willingly gave their time and energy at a difficult time in their lives to join this project and inform others.

Appendix

See Table 1.

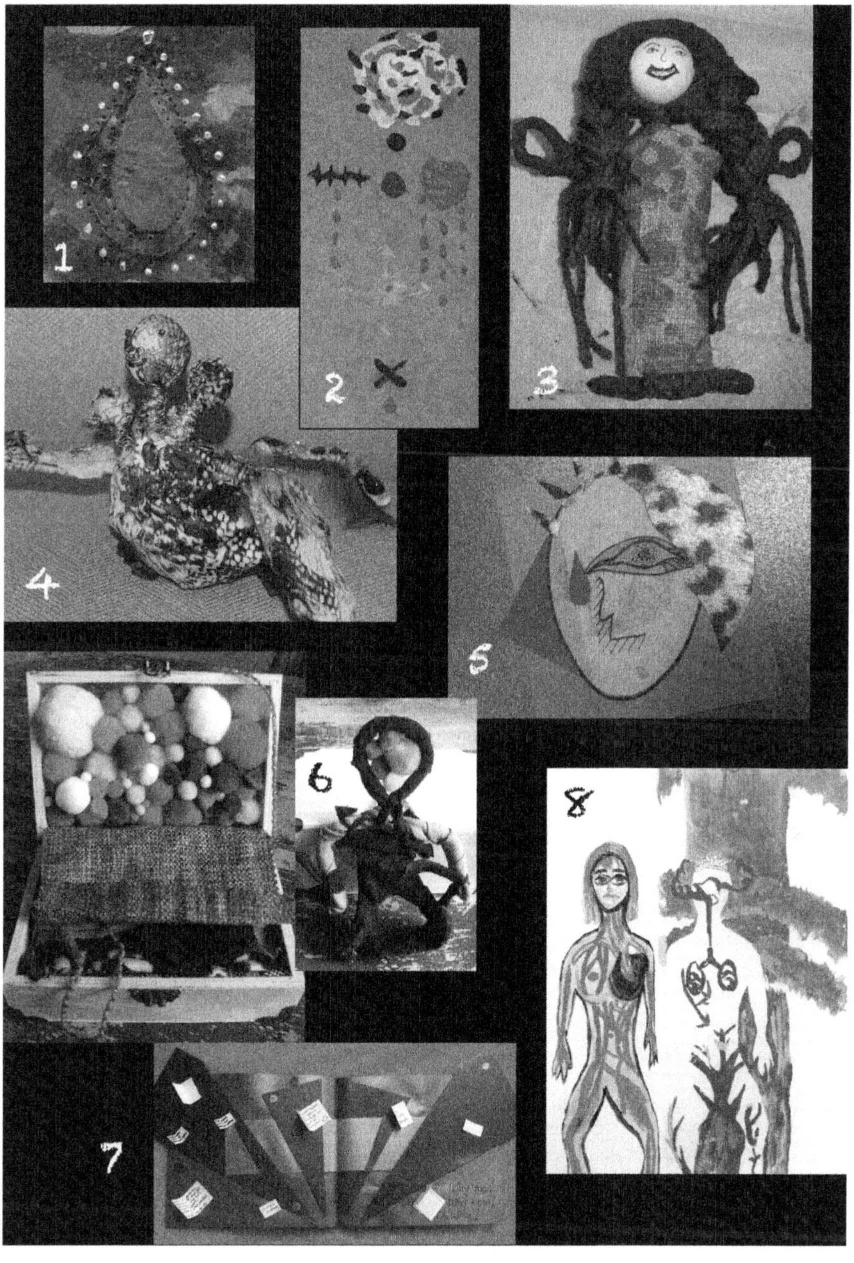

References

Anders, C. K., Johnson, R., Litton, J., Phillips, M., & Bleyer, A. (2009). Breast cancer before age 40 years. *Seminars in Oncology, 36*(3), 237–249.

Bell, S. E. (2006). Living with breast cancer in text and linage: Making art to make sense. *Quality Research in Psychology, 3*(1), 31–44.

Ben-Arye, E., Frenkel, M., Bar-Sela, G., Margalit, R. S., Hermoni, D., & Kuten, A. (2008). Teaching complementary medicine at an academic oncology department. *Journal of Cancer Education, 23*(1), 46–50.

Bennett, J. A., Cameron, L. D., Whitehead, L. C., & Porter, D. (2009). Differences between older and younger cancer survivors in seeking cancer information and using complementary/alternative medicine. *Journal of General Internal Medicine, 24*(10), 1089–1094.

Bocking, Maureen. (2005). A 'don't know' story: art therapy in an NHS medical oncology department. In D. Waller & C. Sibbett (Eds.), *Facing death: Art therapy and cancer care* (pp. 210–222). UK: Open University Press.

Boon, H. S., Olatunde, F., & Zick, S. M. (2007). Trends in complementary/alternative medicine use by breast cancer survivors: Comparing survey data from 1998 and 2005. *BMC Womens Healthy, 7*(4).

Bower, J. E., Meyerowitz, B. E., Desmond, K. A., Bernards, C. A., Rowland, J. H., & Ganz, P. A. (2005). Perceptions of positive meaning and vulnerability following breast cancer: predictors and outcomes among long-term breast cancer survivors. *Annals of Behavioral Medicine, 29*, 236–245.

Breitbart, W., Rosenfeld, B., Gibson, C., Pessin, H., Poppito, S., Nelson, C., et al. (2010). Meaning-centered group psychotherapy for patients with advanced cancer: A pilot randomized controlled trial. *Psycho-Oncology, 19*(1), 21–28.

Canadian Breast Cancer Foundation. (2014). Breast cancer statistics. Retrieved November 2, 2014 from http://www.cbcf.org/central/AboutBreastCancerMain/FactsStats/Pages/Breast-Cancer-Canada.aspx

Canadian Cancer Society. (2010). Cancer in young people. Retrieved November 2, 2014 from http://www.cancer.ca/en/about-us/news/national/2010/cancer-in-young-people/?region=qc#ixzz3HyMzU6Ji

Canadian Cancer Society Statistics. (2009). Retrieved May 7, 2010 from http://www.cancer.ca/Canadawide/About%20cancer/Cancer%20statistics/Stats%20at%20a%20glance/Breast%20cancer.aspx?sc_lang=en

Cancer in Young Adults in Canada. (2006). Cancer Care Ontario http://dsp-psd.pwgsc.gc.ca/Collection/HP5-20-2006E.pdf

Carpenter, J. S., Brockopp, D. Y., & Andrykowski, M. A. (1999). Self-transformation as a factor in the self-esteem and well-being of breast cancer survivors. *Journal of Advanced Nursing, 29* (6), 1402–1411.

Cassileth, B. R., & Deng, G. (2004). Complementary and alternative therapies in cancer. *Oncologist, 9*, 80–89.

Collie, K., Bottorff, J. L., Long, B. C., & Conati, C. (2006a). Distance art groups for women with breast cancer: Guidelines and recommendations. *Supportive Care in Cancer, 14*(8), 849–858.

Collie, K., Bottoroff, J. L., & Long, B. C. (2006b). A narrative view of art therapy and art making by women with breast cancer. *Journal of Health Psychology, 11*, 761–775.

Collie, K., & Long, B. C. (2005). Considering 'meaning' in the context of breast cancer. *Journal of Health Psychology, 10*(6), 843–853.

Complementary Therapies: A Guide for People with Cancer. (2014). Canadian Cancer Society.

Connell, S., Patterson, C., & Newman, B. (2006). A qualitative analysis of reproductive issues raised by young Australian women with breast cancer. *Health Care for Women International, 27*, 94–110.

Davis, C. (2004). Psychosocial needs of women with breast cancer: How can social workers make a difference? *Health and Social Work, 29*(4), 330–334.

Dunn, J., & Steginga, S. K. (2002). Young Women's experience of breast cancer: Defining young and identifying concerns. *Psycho-Oncology, 9*, 137–146.

Gupta, D., Granick, J., Grutsch, J. F., & Lis, C. G. (2007). The prognostic association of health-related quality of life scores with survival in breast cancer. *Supportive Care in Cancer, 4*, 387–393.

Josselson, R., & Lieblich, A. (2003). A framework for narrative research proposals in psychology. In R. Josselson, A. Lieblich, & D. P. McAdams (Eds.), *Up close and personal. The teaching and learning of narrative research* (pp. 259–274). Washington, DC: APA.

Kissane, D. W., Grabsch, B., Clarke, D. M., Smith, G. C., Love, A. W., Bloch, S., et al. (2007). Supportive-expressive group therapy for women with metastatic breast cancer: Survival and psychosocial outcome from a randomized controlled trial. *Psycho-Oncology, 16*, 277–286.

Knobf, M. T. (2007). Psychosocial responses in breast cancer survivors. *Seminars in Oncology Nursing, 23*(1), 71–83.

Landmark, B. T., & Wahl, A. (2002). Living with newly diagnosed breast cancer: A qualitative study of 10 women with newly diagnosed breast cancer. *Journal of Advanced Nursing, 40*(1), 112–121.

Laux, K. (2009). *In her own voice: A narrative inquiry into how three women recently diagnosed with breast cancer utilized the artist's fold book.* Unpublished master's thesis, Concordia University, Montreal, Quebec, Canada.

Lee, V. (2008). The existential plight of cancer: Meaning making as a concrete approach to the intangible search for meaning. *Supportive Care in Cancer, 16*(7), 779–785.

Lee, V., Cohen, S. R., Edgar, L., Laizner, A. M., & Gagnon, A. J. (2006). Meaning-making intervention during breast or colorectal cancer treatment improves self-esteem, optimism, and self-efficacy. *Social Science and Medicine, 62*(12), 3133–3145.

Lee, V., Laux, K., Robitaille, A., Meterissian, S., Gorman, G., & Wexler, S. (2015). Mixed methods and mixed results: lessons learned from research evaluating the impact of group art therapy for women living with breast cancer. Canadian Association of Psychosocial Oncology, Celebrating Leadership in Whole Person Care: CAPO's first 30 years, Montreal, QC, April 22–24, 2015.

Lemieux, J., Maunsell, E., & Provencher, L. (2008). Chemotherapy-induced alopecia and effects on quality of life among women with breast cancer: A literature review. *Psycho-Oncology, 17*(4), 317–328.

Lincoln, Y., & Guba, E. (1985). *Naturalistic inquiry*. Newbury Park, CA: Sage.

Luzzatto, P. (2005). 'Musing with death' in group art therapy with cancer patients. In D. Waller & C. Sibbett (Eds.), *Facing death. Art therapy and cancer care* (pp. 163–171). UK: Open University Press.

Luzzatto, P., & Gabriel, B. (2000). The creative journey: A model for short-term group art therapy with posttreatment cancer patients. *Art Therapy: The Journal of the American Art Therapy Association, 17*(4), 265–269.

Malchiodi, C. A. (Ed.). (1999). *Medical art therapy with adults*. London: Jessica Kingsley.

Marshall, C., & Rossman, G. B. (2006). *Designing qualitative research* (4th ed.). Thousand Oaks, CA: Sage.

Melody. (1995). *Love is in the earth.* Colorado: Earth-Love Publishing House.

Neuman, W. L. (2006). *Social research methods: Qualitative and quantitative approaches* (6th ed.). Boston, MA: Pearson.

Ohlen, J., & Holm, A. K. (2006). Transforming desolation into consolation: Being a mother with life-threatening breast cancer. *Health Care Women International, 27*, 18–44.

Polkinghorne, D. (1988). *Narrative knowing and the human sciences.* New York, NY: State University of New York Press.

Predeger, E. (1996). Womanspirit: A journey into healing through art in breast cancer. *Advances in Nursing Sciences., 18*(3), 48–58.

Richardson, M. A., Sanders, T., Palmer, J. L., Greisinger, A., & Singletary, S. E. (2000). Complementary/Alternative medicine use in a comprehensive cancer center and the implications for oncology. *Journal of Clinical Oncology, 18*(13), 2505–2514.

Serlin, I. A., Classen, C., & Frances, B. (2000). Symposium: Support groups for women with breast cancer: Traditional and alternative expressive approaches. *The Arts in Psychotherapy, 27* (2), 123–138.

Shaha, M., & Bauer-Wu, S. (2009). Early adulthood uprooted transitoriness in young women with breast cancer. *Cancer Nursing, 32*(3), 246–255.

Taylor, E. J. (2000). Transformation of tragedy among women surviving breast cancer. *Oncology Nursing Forum, 27*(5), 781–788.

Turner, J., Kelly, B., & Swanson, C. (2005). Psychosocial impact of newly diagnosed advanced breast cancer. *Psycho-Oncology, 14*(5), 396–407.

Wong-kim, E. C., & Bloom, J. R. (2005). Depression experienced by young women newly diagnosed with breast cancer. *Psycho-Oncology, 14*, 564–573.

Chapter 7
Physical Activity, Locus of Control, and Fear of Recurrence Among Cancer Survivors from a Community-Based Cancer Support Program

Roxana Mititelu, Achuthan Aruljothy and Tanya R. Fitzpatrick

Introduction

This pilot study aims to examine the relationship between physical activity, locus of control (LOC), and fear of recurrence among participants in a community cancer support program. With the advent of newer and more effective treatments, many people find themselves metamorphosing into their new identity as a cancer survivor. This new identity brings the lingering fear of recurrence, which may negatively impact the survivor's quality of life. It is thus necessary for health-care practitioners to examine the association between LOC and physical activity as a means of possibly reducing and lessening the negative effects of fear of recurrence.

Simard and Savard (2009) define fear of cancer recurrence as the fear or worry of the possibility that the cancer will return or progress in the same organ or in another part of the body. LOC is defined as a psychological construct predicting that cognitive structural expectations influence behavioral and emotional states (Farone et al. 2007). In other words, LOC refers to the individual's belief that their behavior, or more specifically, the reinforcements from their behavior, is ascribed to personal (internal locus) or situational (external locus) elements, thereby suggesting that an internal LOC may have some influence on the experience of fear of cancer recurrence (Watson et al. 1990). Physical activities, viewed as a positive intervention, are

R. Mititelu (✉) · A. Aruljothy
Faculty of Medicine, McGill University, 3655 Sir William Osler, Montreal, QC H3G 1Y6, Canada
e-mail: roxana.mititelu@mail.mcgill.ca

A. Aruljothy
e-mail: achuthan.aruljothy@mail.mcgill.ca

T.R. Fitzpatrick
Department of Nursing, McGill University, 449 Mount Pleasant Ave, Westmount, QC H3Y 3G9, Canada
e-mail: tanya.fitzpatrick@asu.edu

T.R. Fitzpatrick (ed.), *Treating Vulnerable Populations of Cancer Survivors: A Biopsychosocial Approach*, DOI 10.1007/978-3-319-32364-0_7

part of leisure, recreational, household, work-related activities, as well as exercise programs (Coronado et al. 2011). Physical activity is described as intentional body movement, as opposed to exercise, which refers to purposeful efforts to augment activity beyond the bare minimum required to perform social roles (Wagner et al. 1992). With the advances of screening, improvements on diagnoses, and novel treatments, the length of time between the diagnosis and eventual death has greatly prolonged, emphasizing the importance of studying the survivorship in this population. Cancer is a multifaceted disease creating many hurdles for those it touches. It affects not only the person with the diagnosis but it impacts caregivers in terms of quality of life, financial costs, and more widely it is a public health burden (Brown et al. 2001). Therefore, as oncology professionals, it is imperative to help and guide survivors and their caregivers to provide methods to manage this fear and preserve their quality of life.

Literature Review

Fear of Recurrence Among Cancer Survivors

In 2012, there were more than 13 million cancer survivors in the United States. By 2022, this number is expected to increase to approximately 18 million (Siegel et al. 2012). Studies have shown that cancer survivors report fear of recurrence as a major concern irrespective of their cultural background or cancer type (Ashing Giwa et al. 2004; Ferrell et al. 1995; Matthews 2003; Mullens et al. 2004; Skaali et al. 2009). Furthermore, the fear of recurrence is pervasive and persists in patients for long periods of time, even after the initial diagnosis and treatment (Humphris et al. 2003; Lee-Jones et al. 1997; Welch-McCaffrey et al. 1989). Baker et al. (2005) found that despite surviving a year past diagnosis, more than two-thirds of cancer patients experienced fear of cancer recurrence, with more than half being fearful about the future. This study also found that among cancer survivors of the most prevalent cancers (i.e., breast, prostate, and colorectal, lung), fear of recurrence was either their primary or secondary concern. In a breast cancer study, women shared how pervasive the fear of recurrence was, with even minor medical symptoms unrelated to cancer (e.g., spider bite) triggering the fear of recurrence (Ferrell et al. 1997). Moreover, fear of recurrence is not only a universal concern throughout survivorship, it has also been linked to poorer psychological adjustment, increased emotional distress, and lower quality of life outcomes (Stanton et al. 2002; Vickberg 2003). A study constructed by Stefanek et al. (1989) demonstrated that the high degree of worry in cancer survivors negatively affected their daily routine and interpersonal relationships.

Factors that may have a relationship to fear of recurrence are age, education, and gender. It has been shown that younger age, more education, and female gender potentially augment the fear of recurrence (Davis-Ali et al. 1993; Gil et al. 2004;

Stanton et al. 2003). Some studies suggest that fear of recurrence is not only widespread among cancer survivors, but its effects can be detrimental to the outcome of the patient already facing much adversity (Lee-Jones et al. 1997). It is thus imperative to examine possible interventions to mediate the negative impact of fear of cancer recurrences and assess its relationship to LOC and physical activity.

Locus of Control and Fear of Recurrence Among Cancer Survivors

Rotter (1966) first proposed the psychological concept of LOC as a measure of predicting the effect of one's cognitive expectations on one's behavior and emotional state. Furthermore, LOC attributes whether a personal element (internal locus) or situational element (external locus) influences a person's behavior. Most notably, LOC has been implicated as a stress mediator (Watson et al. 1990). A sense of personal control or an internal LOC has been associated with positive health, well-being, and a positive adjustment to cancer, positive coping, and cancer-related health behaviors (Thompson and Spacapan 1991; Farone et al. 2007; Taylor 1983; Taylor and Brown 1994; Watson et al. 1990). Bundek et al. (1993) demonstrate an internal LOC correlated positively with the likelihood of performing breast self-examination, while correlating negatively with Pap test screening behaviors.

In general, studies examining LOC among cancer survivors have resulted in conflicting conclusions. Some recent studies have shown that an internal LOC has been correlated with positive affect, and lower rates of depression in cancer survivors (Knappe and Pinquart 2009; Naus et al. 2005). In contrast, a literature review regarding psychosocial factors found that LOC only had a minor predictive effect on the prognosis of cancer (Garssen 2004). Furthermore, De Boer et al. (1999) found no association between loci of control and relapse or survival rates. These studies did not, however, specifically address the role LOC plays and the fear of recurrence, although it would seem that the LOC might assist in managing the fear of recurrence.

The presence of disputing results regarding the relationship between LOC and cancer can be theoretically explained by the extent to which one's beliefs correspond to 'reality'. A study examining LOC and depression noted that participants who perceived themselves to have some control had less symptoms of depression, regardless of how realistic their beliefs were (Taylor 1983). Following these results Taylor (1983) hypothesized that in certain circumstance such as major illnesses which one has limited control over, a degree of self-deception can have a positive effect on adaptation and coping. Andrykowski and Brady (1994) led further analysis of this concept to examine the interplay of locus control in different contexts of reality by comparing the effects of the beliefs among people with diagnoses of differing severity, and among those who had and who had not experienced prior treatment failure. The results of this study found differing responses that correlated to the person's LOC such that for those with a strong internal LOC, the severity of the diagnosis was a predictor of distress but prior treatment failure was not. For those with a strong external LOC, both severity of risk and prior treatment failure predicted distress. Therefore, based on Wheaton's (1985) direct effect model of stress reduction, LOC can be seen as a form of social support possibly mediating the negative effects of fear of recurrence.

Physical Activity and Fear of Recurrence Among Cancer Survivors

Physical activity has widespread positive effects among cancer survivors, improving symptoms, physiologic effects, vigor, and cardiorespiratory fitness after cancer treatment (Dimeo et al. 1999; Schmitz et al. 2005). Data from a recent study with almost 3000 breast cancer survivors showed that high levels of post-treatment physical activity was associated with a 26–40 % reduction in the risk of breast cancer recurrence, breast cancer-specific mortality, and all-cause mortality (Holmes et al. 2005). This reduction was seen with as little as 1–3 h per week of moderate intensity activity (Holmes et al. 2005). Similar associations between physical activity and colorectal cancer survivors have been shown (Meyerhardt et al. 2006; Schwartz 2004). There are few studies that have specifically analyzed physical activity and fear of recurrence; however, a study by Young and White (2006) showed that higher levels of fear of recurrence are correlated with lower levels of physical activity thus resulting in increased fatigue, and decreased quality of life. As shown, few studies have analyzed the relationship between fear of recurrence, physical activity, and LOC.

Theoretical Perspectives

Wheaton (1985) suggests that social support is positively associated with psychological well-being and physical health via the direct effect model. The model suggests that a person's baseline vulnerability to experience stress is the result of a stressful exposure or situation. The stress can then be dissipated, used for conflict resolution, or the stress can be effectively coped with so as to reduce the deleterious physical and emotional effects that result from lingering stress. Social and physical supports, which are described by Wheaton as any internal or external resources that facilitate effective coping, play a key role in mediating the effect of stress by acting directly to reduce it. Conceptually, increasing levels of fear of recurrence are associated with increasing levels of stress, with physical activity and LOC being forms of social support, acting as buffers. The hypothesis suggests that buffers,

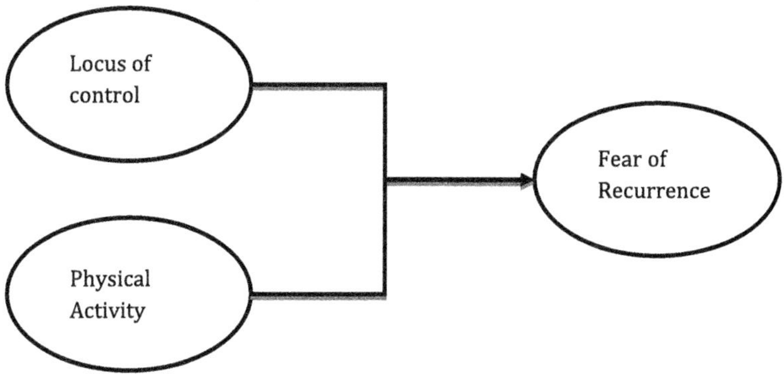

Fig. 1 The direct effect model as proposed by Wheaton (1985)

different forms of social support, mediate stressful life situations and diminishes the impact the stressful experience has on the person. Both physical activity and LOC can be seen as types of social support, and thus the type and quality of support a cancer survivor receives may affect their adjustment and their fear of recurrence.

Figure 1 represents the Direct Effect Model as proposed by Wheaton (1985).

Summary of the Literature

The overwhelming majority of research shows that fear of recurrence plays a key role in negatively impacting the quality of life among cancer survivors (Humphris et al. 2003; Gil et al. 2004; Farone et al. 2005). Research concerning physical activity and LOC suggest that the potential supportive role the two constructs may have on a stressful situation. Although the presented studies are a key to creating a knowledge base for survivorship post-cancer diagnosis, they point to the need for further research. The direct effect model (Wheaton 1985) also posits that a potential relationship can be seen between physical activity, LOC, and a stressful life event such as the fear of cancer recurring. Few studies have examined the relationship between physical activity, LOC, and the fear of recurrence among cancer survivors. This current study highlights the importance of addressing the negative impact of fear of recurrence, which is critical to living and coping with a diagnosis of cancer.

Hypothesis

With increasing lengths of survival, factors negatively affecting cancer survivors become increasingly important. Fear of recurrence is pervasive and long lasting. Pain and limitations on daily activities due to fear, and recovery from surgery impede one's ability to enjoy life's activities and to feel independent. Previous researches regarding LOC and physical activity have been shown to have positive outcomes on quality of life among cancer survivors (Andrykowski and Brady 1994; Meyerhardt et al. 2006). It is therefore hypothesized, based on the literature and the theoretical perspectives from the direct effect model (Wheaton 1985) that physical activity and LOC will have a modifying effect on the negative impact of fear of recurrence among cancer survivors (Farone et al. 2005).

Methodology

Site and Data

The data for this study was based on participants from a community cancer support program located in Beaconsfield, Quebec. As of December 2013, the cancer support program served 899 participants in this region (WICWC this October 2013 statistics, Unpublished manuscript). The cancer support program used in this study offers a variety of services using an integrated approach to wellness, spanning from support groups for caregivers, psychological education, peer-support groups, to support groups for newly diagnosed patients. Additionally, the center offers an open gym with a personal trainer, yoga, nutritional cooking classes, art classes, meditation, Qi Gong, Reiki, therapeutic touch, and reflexology. The services offered by the wellness center or cancer support program are free and can be used by anyone from the time of their diagnosis until 1-year of post-treatment.

Sample

The sample for this study was based on cancer survivors having a variety of cancer types with breast cancer being the most common. Approximately 38 % of the participants being survivors of breast cancer, 48 % of participants with active cancer, and 39 % of the participants have a metastatic cancer (WICWC this October 2013 statistics, Unpublished manuscript). The majority of the participants ranged from 46 to 60 years old at the time of diagnosis and an overwhelming majority were female (78 %).

Data Collection

Initial consent approval for the study was provided by an affiliated Montreal hospital and was approved by the executive director of the cancer support program. The executive director distributed information regarding the study to all the participants at the community cancer support program. The research associates went to the center on a previously scheduled date to distribute the questionnaires. The participants were provided with an informed consent form and were ensured complete confidentiality. The consent form was developed and approved by the director of the center before being administered. If the participants agreed to participate they were provided with the questionnaires for the study which took approximately 30 min to complete, and were then collected by the research associates. The research associates went to the community wellness center to distribute the questionnaires and collected them the same day. The entire questionnaire and informed consent were also translated into French for French-speaking participants.

Measurement of Variables

Dependent variable: Fear of cancer recurrence. The dependent variable of fear of recurrence was measured using a modified version of the fear of cancer recurrence inventory (FCRI) (Simard and Savard 2009). The function of the inventory is to assess an individual's fear of cancer recurrence, based on several dimensions and factors. The FCRI is comprised of seven factors: triggers, severity, psychological distress, coping strategies, functional impairment, insight, and reassurance. Each question is scored on a scale of 0–4; 0 represents never and 4 represents all the time.

The first factor, *triggers*, consists of eight items of which seven evaluate particular scenarios that evoke the possibility of a cancer recurrence and one item to assess the degree of avoidance for potential fear of cancer recurrence. The second factor, *severity*, consists of nine items that evaluate "the presence, the frequency, the intensity, and the duration of the thoughts associated with FCR, the perceived risk of recurrence, the legitimacy of worrying about cancer recurrence, and the presence of other unpleasant thoughts or images that come to mind in association with FCR" (Simard and Savard 2009). Moreover, it includes one reverse item evaluating the thought that one is cured. The third factor, *psychological distress*, is comprised of emotions evoked by cancer recurrence thoughts. An example of a psychological distress question is "*When I think about the possibility of cancer recurrence, I feel… Worry, fear or anxiety*". The fourth factor, *functional impairments*, involves assessing the extent of functional impairment, such as "*My thoughts or fears about the possibility of cancer disrupt…. My state of mind or my mood*". The fifth factor, *insight*, consists of three items evaluating the degree to which individuals interpret their fear as excessive or unreasonable. The response to "*My thoughts or fears about the possibility of cancer recurrence disrupt… I feel that I worry excessively about the possibility of cancer recurrence*" is used to assess their insight. The sixth factor, *reassurance,* ascertains reassurance behaviors particular to fear of cancer recurrence. "*When I think about the possibility of cancer recurrence, I use the following strategies to reassure myself… I call my doctor or other health professional*". The seventh factor, *coping strategies*, consists of certain strategies that may be used to cope with cancer recurrence, by asking "*When I think about the possibility of cancer recurrence, I use the following strategies to reassure myself... I pray, meditate or do relaxation*".

Independent Variables

Physical activities. The independent variable of physical activity was measured using the compendium of physical activity using the metabolic equivalency tasks (METs) as the base unit (Ainsworth et al. 1993) for the purpose of validating physical activity. The research associates used METs scores to assess a comprehensive list of specific activities performed at the center in addition to activities executed at home or in the community. All activities are assigned a unit based on their rate of energy expenditure expressed as METs. METs measure the hours/week to assess the energy cost of physical activities and are defined as the ratio of metabolic rate (rate of energy consumption) during a specific physical activity. For example, at the wellness center yoga is given 4 METs units while walking at a normal pace is 3 METs units.

Locus of control. The second major independent variable was measured using the locus of control questionnaire based on Rotter's (1966) generalized expectancies for internal versus external control of reinforcement. Our study used the brief scale to determine the participants' LOC. An example question is "When I make plans, I am almost certain that I can make them work". The participants respond on a scale of 1–5 with 1 referring to strongly disagree and 5 referring to strongly agree. The higher the score the more a participant's' LOC is internal signifying a belief that the person believes their choices influences behavioral outcomes. A lower score denotes an external locus, thus referring to a person's belief that outcomes in their life are governed by an external power out of their control.

Control Variables

To assist in clarifying the relationship between the major variables in the study, control variables were included such as age, gender, education, marital status, type of cancer, type of treatment (i.e., chemotherapy, radiation, and surgery), length of time since diagnosis, and previous cancer recurrences. These variables were included in the self-reported questionnaire. They were measured as follows: age was measured as three categorical dummy variables; less than 44 years of age, 45–64 years of age, and 65 years of age or older, and coded as 1 = Yes; 0 = No. The other control variables, such as gender (male, female), marital status (married/common law partnership or not married), and type of treatment (chemotherapy, radiation, surgery), were measured as categorical dummy variables, and coded as 1 = yes and 0 = no. The variable, education, was also coded as a dummy variable, with the categories being: high school, undergraduate, and graduate/postgraduate in which, 1 = yes and 0 = no.

In particular, age, education, and gender have been associated with fear of recurrence (Davis-Ali et al. 1993; Gil et al. 2004; Stanton et al. 2003). Among personal factors, it has been shown that younger age, higher education, and female gender contribute to fear of recurrence (Bowman et al. 2003). Gil et al. (2004) concluded that more educated women had more triggers about recurrence than less educated women. Additionally, female cancer survivors have reported more fear of recurrence than male survivors (Davis-Ali et al. 1993). Since previous research demonstrates that age, education, and gender interact with fear of recurrence, our study controlled for these factors as to remove any confounding effects.

Data Analysis

The data were examined using the SPSS 11.01 statistical software program. A correlation matrix to initially examine the relationship between all the major variables was conducted. Regression analysis using the direct effect model in Model 1 (Wheaton 1985; Tran et al. 1996) examined the effects of the control variables of age, gender, marital status, education, radiation therapy, surgery and hormone therapy on the total summary score of Fear of Recurrence. Subsequently, Model 2 examined the direct effects of the control variables plus adding physical activity (METs) on Fear of Recurrence. Model 3 examined the direct effects of the control variables and LOC on fear of recurrence. Finally, Model 4 regressed the control variables with the independent variables of physical activity and LOC on the fear of recurrence. Finally, we repeated the linear regression using the same above-mentioned models on each component of the fear of recurrence items, which includes triggers, severity, psychological distress, functioning impairments, insight, reassurance, and coping strategies.

Results

Demographics

The demographic information describing the total population of cancer survivors is presented in Table 1 (N = 32). Ninety-one percent of the participants were female. Average education was college or postsecondary education (75 %). Approximately 72 % were married. The average age was between 45 and 64 years (72 %). Of the 32 individuals constituting the sample, 50 % had breast cancer, 12.5 % had uterine or other gynecological cancer. With regards to their time of diagnosis, 87.5 % of the study population were diagnosed after January 1, 2011, with 91 % of them having no prior cancer recurrence. Moreover, 91 % of the individuals in the study were currently participating in physical activity.

Table 1 Demographic data for the total sample of cancer survivors ($N = 32$)

	N	%	Valid %
Age			
0–45 years	5	15.6	
45–64 years	23	71.9	
65+ years	4	12.5	
Gender			
Male	3	9.4	
Female	29	90.6	
Marital status			
Not married	9	28.1	
Married, common law	23	71.9	
Education[a]			
High school	7	21.9	22.6
College	24	75.0	77.4
Type of cancer			
Breast	16	50.0	
Prostate	1	3.1	
Colorectal	2	6.3	
Gynecological	4	12.5	
Other	9	28.1	
Time of diagnosis[a]			
Before January 1, 2011	3	9.4	9.7
After January 1, 2011	28	87.5	90.3
Previous recurrence			
No	29	90.6	
Yes	3	9.4	
Treatment			
Chemotherapy	23	71.9	
Radiation	19	59.4	
Surgery	25	78.1	
Hormonal therapy	11	34.4	
Other treatment	5	15.6	
Current participation in physical activity			
No	3	9.4	
Yes	29	90.6	

Note [a]The *N*s may not equal 32 due to missing data

Correlation Matrix

A correlation matrix was performed to initially examine the relationship between all the variables. The results revealed that several control variables plus physical activities (METs) were significantly related to the dependent variable of fear of recurrence. For example, participation in physical activity, having surgery, and prostate cancer were significantly related to coping, which is one of the items representing fear of recurrence. Following this, LOC was related to having surgery, and surgery was also related to impairment. A complete description of the initial relationships between the variables can be made available upon request.

Regression Analyses

Physical Activity, Locus of Control, and Fear of Recurrence

The results of the regression analyzing the effects of LOC, physical activity and the control variables on the fear of recurrence indicate that LOC and physical activity were not significantly related to the total summary score of fear of recurrence.

Physical Activity, Locus of Control, and Impairment

Table 2 presents the results of the regression analyses examining the effects of physical activity, LOC, and the control variables on the specific item of impairment representing fear of recurrence. The results reveal that having surgery as a treatment is associated with less functional impairment, suggesting that cancer survivors experienced less functional impairment post surgical interventions. Specifically, having undergone surgery may result in less psychological and physical impairment ($b = -6.99$; p-value < 0.05). The remainder of the control variables was not significantly related to impairment. The total variance for this model explained by control variables, physical activity, and LOC on impairment was $r^2 = 0.40$.

Physical Activity, Locus of Control, and Coping

Table 3 presents the results of the regression analyses examining the effects of physical activity, LOC, and the control variables on the specific item of coping representing fear of recurrence. The results reveal that education had a significant relationship with coping suggesting that more educated cancer survivors were more likely to cope better with their illness ($b = 8.45$; p-value < 0.05). Additionally,

Table 2 Regression analysis using control variables, locus of control and physical activity on the fear of recurrence ($N = 32$)

Variable	Fear of recurrence		
	b	SE	*B*
Age	10.56	12.41	0.21
Gender	18.30	20.59	0.21
Martial	15.14	12.92	0.26
Education	20.34	14.57	0.33
Chemotherapy	20.71	12.56	0.37
Radiation	7.42	11.63	0.14
Surgery	−4.77	15.39	−0.07
Hormone	−7.90	11.99	−0.15
METs	0.00	0.05	0.02
LOC	−0.80	1.69	−0.11
r^2	0.22		

Note $^*p < 0.05$, $^{**}p < 0.01$, $^{***}p < 0.001$ two-tailed test

LOC was also significantly related to coping, in that individuals who had a higher score of LOC were more likely to have better coping skills ($b = 0.03$; $p < 0.05$). The total variance for this model explained by the control variables, physical activity, and LOC on coping was $r^2 = 0.49$. Moreover, the other components of fear of recurrence were analyzed for any significant relationship with the independent variables and these results did not reach statistical significance. The results of these analyses can be made available upon request to the author.

Table 3 Regression analyses of control variables, locus of control and physical activity on impairment and coping ($N = 32$)

Variable	Impairment			Coping		
	b	SE	*B*	*b*	SE	*B*
Age	3.89	2.62	0.32	−4.71	3.20	−0.29
Gender	2.86	4.36	0.14	−3.67	5.32	−0.13
Martial	5.50	2.73	0.39	−2.01	3.34	−0.11
Education	1.87	3.08	0.13	8.45*	3.76	0.43
Chemotherapy	4.12	2.66	0.30	3.52	3.24	0.20
Radiation	−1.44	2.46	−0.11	−0.60	3.00	−0.04
Surgery	−6.99*	3.26	−0.45	7.65	3.97	0.37
Hormone	−1.68	2.54	−0.13	−0.79	3.10	−0.05
METs	−0.01	0.01	−0.16	0.52	0.44	0.22
LOC	−0.19	0.36	−0.11	0.03*	0.01	0.43
r^2	0.40				0.49	

Note $^*p < 0.05$, $^{**}p < 0.01$, $^{***}p < 0.001$ two-tailed test

Discussion

This study examined the relationship between physical activity, LOC, and fear of cancer recurrence among participants in a community cancer support program. Using the direct effect model (Wheaton 1985), it was hypothesized that LOC and physical activity conceptualized as means of social support could lessen the negative effects of fear of recurrence. The results of this study provide support for the direct effect model by revealing that cancer survivors who had higher levels of education and higher scores of LOC were able to cope more effectively, a key component to lessening the fear of recurrence. Also the results show that undergoing surgery is associated with less functional impairment, another key component of fear of recurrence.

Interestingly, previous studies have shown that education levels tend to contribute to a greater fear of recurrence (Bowman et al. 2003; Gil et al. 2004). While more recent studies have shown the opposite result, higher education levels tend to result in the lessening of the fear of recurrence (Hart et al. 2008; Koch et al. 2013). However, in our study, education had no significant relationship to the fear of recurrence but was related to coping, a component of fear of recurrence. Specifically, higher education levels were significantly related to one's ability to psychologically cope with the fear of cancer recurrence. Highly educated individuals may possess a greater comprehension and rationalization of their cancer diagnosis thus potentially lessening any fears. The results emphasize the complicated nature of fear of recurrence with many components interacted upon by multitude of factors constituting cancer survivorship.

Additionally, a survivor's perceived LOC, specifically a greater internal LOC, was associated with a greater ability to cope with the fear of cancer recurrence. Rotter's (1966) model predicts a high score of LOC is related to greater awareness of autonomy and control of one's behavior. Thus, possibly the association between an internal LOC and coping exists due to a person's autonomy to seek out methods to cope with their fear of recurrence. For example, survivors with a higher internal LOC possibly seek out more coping activities such as yoga, tai chi, and other physical activities; thus experiencing less fear of recurrence.

This study reveals a significant relationship between surgical intervention and the impairment component of fear of recurrence. Based on the results, it is suggested that undergoing surgery, as opposed to chemotherapy or radiation therapy, is a singular phenomenon that is associated with fewer functional sequelae. This can be explained possibly by the advent of minimally invasive procedures, such as laparoscopy or in the context of breast cancer partial mastectomies, where the physical outcomes are less invasive thus resulting in less physical impairment and cognitive impairment. Previous studies have shown that patients undergoing chemotherapy experience cognitive impairment or "chemobrain" which impairs quality of life, and is associated with a decrease in physical activity (Fitch et al. 2008; Littman et al. 2010).

Conclusions

The purpose of this pilot study was to examine the relationship between physical activity, LOC, and fear of recurrence among participants in a community cancer support program. The results support the theories of social support as proposed in the direct effect model where LOC and physical activity are seen as social supports having a moderating effect on the negative impact of fear of recurrence (Wheaton 1985). Specific results from this pilot study indicate that a stronger internal LOC is related to better coping when faced with the fear of cancer recurring. Additionally, those with higher education levels also experience better coping. Finally, undergoing a surgical treatment is related to less functional impairment which is also related to the fear of recurrence.

Implications for Clinical Practice

This study suggests that physical activity and LOC are therapeutic interventions that can mediate the negative effect of fear of recurrence for cancer survivors to a certain degree. Physical activity is a form of social support with a great potential of lessening the constant dread and fear of cancer recurrence via participation in physical activity programs and facilities directed toward cancer-related community interventions (Leimanis and Fitzpatrick 2014; Wheaton 1985). Fear of recurrence is a chronic anxiety plaguing cancer survivors, and health-care practitioners can alleviate it by reinforcing the health benefits of a strong LOC through an allied relationship based on mutual trust, respect, and empowerment of their own health. LOC can be strengthened by encouraging patient autonomy and by providing a voice to survivor and their experience. As health-care practitioners become aware of the experience of the fear of cancer recurrence, they can then promote available physical activity resources in the community to assist in addressing the quality of life of cancer survivors. Furthermore, health-care practitioners can empower survivors by strengthening patient autonomy via providing choices in their treatment and therapeutic plan and by acknowledging the daily challenges of the cancer survivorship experience. The results of this study associating LOC and fear of recurrence provide further support for additional interventions to address personal coping skills, which can have a mitigating effect on fear of recurrence (Leimanis and Fitzpatrick 2014; Wheaton 1985). Armed with this knowledge, health-care practitioner including physicians, nurses, social workers, and other oncology professionals can proactively improve the quality of life of cancer survivors by encouraging physical activity and nurturing an internal locus control through patient autonomy.

Implication for Future Research

Given the results, additional research is necessitated to further elucidate the different factors impacting fear of recurrence. Individual case studies analyzing the fear of recurrence are warranted since the concept is global, though the experience of fear of recurrence during survivorship is an individual experience for many people. Additional research may further capture the individual concept of fear of recurrence by using a qualitative research design to also explore the essence of the meaning of fear using the individuals personnel statements.

Limitations

Several limitations of the study are warranted. The study sample used only one cancer support program providing a limited sample size, thus making it difficult to generalize the results to the larger population of participants using physical activities at other community cancer support programs. However, the importance of the results from this study are useful for guiding future explorations and replications when examining fear of recurrence with larger populations of cancer survivors. In addition, the sample was heterogeneous and did not include the stage of the cancer and disease progression (local versus metastasized), which would no doubt have an influence on an individual's fear of recurrence, LOC, and possibly affect the individual's ability to participate in physical activities. The study used a self-reported questionnaire assessing physical activities through the compendium of physical activity using the METs (Ainsworth et al. 1993). Although this measure is used widely in studies, the questionnaire may have resulted in an under- or over-reporting of the participants' number and frequency of physical activity participation. The METs scoring can range from 0.9 (sleeping) to 18 (running speed at 17.5 km/h), and are dependent on an individual's resting metabolic rate (RMR), which in itself depends on lean body mass, as opposed to total weight (Ainsworth et al. 1993; Leimanis and Fitzpatrick 2014). Furthermore, the fear of recurrence is a complex experience involving many spheres of a survivor's life (Simard and Savard 2009). The FCRI, despite being one of the only validated questionnaires measuring the concept, may be limited in capturing the individual aspects not included in the questionnaire.

However, the results of this pilot study demonstrate the necessity of interventions designed to foster and nurture an internal LOC and to promote increased participation in physical activity as they relate to the decrease fear of recurrence and by doing so increase the quality of life for cancer survivors. Fear of recurrence is a process that occurs from the onset of diagnosis, during survivorship and continues to be a source of anxiety for the patients. With prolonged survival rates, the cancer survivorship journey necessitates ongoing attention by health-care practitioners as to improve the quality of life of this important vulnerable population.

Acknowledgements The authors wish to gratefully acknowledge the assistance and support from the staff at Hope and Cope Cancer Support Program and the staff at West Island Cancer Wellness Center particularly the director Deborah Magwood. Please direct all the correspondence to the first author, Roxana Mititelu, Faculty of Medicine, McGill University, Roxana.mititelu@mail.mcgill.ca, 514-743-7724.

References

Ainsworth, B. E., Haskell, W. L., Leon, A. S., Jacobs, D. R., Montoye, H. J., Sallis, J. F., & Paffenbarger, R. S. (1993). Compendium of physical activities: Classification of energy costs of human physical activities. *Medicine and Science in Sports and Exercise, 25*, 71.

Andrykowski, M. A., & Brady, M. J. (1994). Health locus of control and psychological distress in cancer patients: Interactive effects of context. *Journal of Behavioral Medicine, 17*(5), 439–458.

Ashing Giwa, K. T., Padilla, G., Tejero, J., Kraemer, J., Wright, K., Coscarelli, A., & Hills, D. (2004). Understanding the breast cancer experience of women: A qualitative study of African American, Asian American, Latina and Caucasian cancer survivors. *Psycho-Oncology, 13*(6), 408–428.

Baker, F., Denniston, M., Smith, T., & West, M. M. (2005). Adult cancer survivors: how are they faring?. *Cancer, 104*(S11), 2565–2576.

Bowman, K. F., Deimling, G. T., Smerglia, V., Sage, P., & Kahana, B. (2003). Appraisal of the cancer experience by older long-term survivors. *Psycho-Oncology, 12*(3), 226–238.

Brown, M. L., Lipscomb, J., & Snyder, C. (2001). The burden of illness of cancer: economic cost and quality of life 1. *Annual Review of Public Health, 22*(1), 91–113.

Bundek, N. I., Marks, G., & Richardson, J. L. (1993). Role of health locus of control beliefs in cancer screening of elderly Hispanic women. *Health Psychology, 12*(3), 193.

Coronado, G. D., Sos, C., Talbot, J., Do, H. H., & Taylor, V. M. (2011). To be healthy and to live long, we have to exercise: Psychosocial factors related to physical activity among Cambodian Americans. *Journal of Community Health, 36*, 381–388.

Davis-Ali, S. H., Chesler, M. A., & Chesney, B. K. (1993). Recognizing cancer as a family disease: Worries and support reported by patients and spouses. *Social Work in Health Care, 19* (2), 45–65.

De Boer, M., Ryckman, R., Pruyn, J., & Van den Borne, H. (1999). Psychosocial correlates of cancer relapse and survival: A literature review. *Patient Education and Counseling, 37*(3), 215–230.

Dimeo, F. C., Stieglitz, R., Novelli-Fischer, U., Fetscher, S., & Keul, J. (1999). Effects of physical activity on the fatigue and psychologic status of cancer patients during chemotherapy. *Cancer, 85*(10), 2273–2277.

Farone, D. W., Fitzpatrick, T. R., & Bushfield, S. Y. (2007). Hope, locus of control, and quality of health among elder Latina cancer survivors. *Social Work in Health Care, 46*(2), 51–70.

Farone, D. W., Fitzpatrick, T. R., & Tran, T. V. (2005). Use of senior centers as a moderator of stress-related distress among Latino elders. *Journal of Gerontological Social Work, 46*(1), 65–83.

Ferrell, B. R., Dow, K. H., Leigh, S., Ly, J., & Gulasekaram, P. (1995). *Quality of life in long-term cancer survivors* (Vol. 22, No. 6, p. 915). Paper presented at the Oncology Nursing Forum.

Ferrell, B. R., Grant, M. M., Funk, B., Otis-Green, S., & Garcia, N. (1997). Quality of life in breast cancer survivors as identified by focus groups. *Psycho-Oncology, 6*(1), 13–23.

Fitch, M. I., Armstrong, J., & Tsang, S. (2008). Patients' experiences with cognitive changes after chemotherapy. *Canadian Oncology Nursing Journal, 18*(4), 180–192.

Garssen, B. (2004). Psychological factors and cancer development: Evidence after 30 years of research. *Clinical Psychology Review, 24*(3), 315–338.

Gil, K. M., Mishel, M. H., Belyea, M., Germino, B., Porter, L. S., Carlton LaNey, I., & Stewart, J. (2004). *Triggers of uncertainty about recurrence and long-term treatment side effects in older African American and Caucasian breast cancer survivors* (Vol. 31, No. 3, pp. 633–639). Paper presented at the Oncology Nursing Forum.

Hart, S. L., Latini, D. M., Cowan, J. E., Carroll, P. R., & CaPSURE™ Investigators. (2008). Fear of recurrence, treatment satisfaction, and quality of life after radical prostatectomy for prostate cancer. *Supportive Care in Cancer, 16*(2), 161–169.

Holmes, M. D., Chen, W. Y., Feskanich, D., Kroenke, C. H., & Colditz, G. A. (2005). Physical activity and survival after breast cancer diagnosis. *JAMA: The Journal of the American Medical Association, 293*(20), 2479–2486.

Humphris, G., Rogers, S., McNally, D., Lee-Jones, C., Brown, J., & Vaughan, D. (2003). Fear of recurrence and possible cases of anxiety and depression in orofacial cancer patients. *International Journal of Oral and Maxillofacial Surgery, 32*(5), 486–491.

Knappe, S., & Pinquart, M. (2009). Tracing criteria of successful aging health, locus of control, and well-being in older patients with internal diseases. *Psychology, Health & Medicine, 14*(2), 201–212.

Koch, L., Jansen, L., Brenner, H., & Arndt, V. (2013). Fear of recurrence and disease progression in long-term (≥ 5 years) cancer survivors—A systematic review of quantitative studies. *Psycho-Oncology, 22*(1), 1–11.

Lee-Jones, C., Humphris, G., Dixon, R., & Bebbington Hatcher, M. (1997). Fear of cancer recurrence—A literature review and proposed cognitive formulation to explain exacerbation of recurrence fears. *Psycho-Oncology, 6*(2), 95–105.

Leimanis, M. L., & Fitzpatrick, T. R. (2014). Physical activities and distress among participants of a Cancer Wellness Centre: A community-based pilot study. *International Journal of Physics Medicine & Rehabilitation, 2*(193), 1000. doi:10.4172/2329-9096.193.

Littman, A. J., Tang, M.-T., & Rossing, M. A. (2010). Longitudinal study of recreational physical activity in breast cancer survivors. *Journal of Cancer Survivorship, 4*, 119–127.

Matthews, A. B. (2003). *Role and gender differences in cancer-related distress: A comparison of survivor and caregiver self-reports* (Vol. 30, No. 3, pp. 493–499). Paper presented at the Oncology Nursing Forum.

Meyerhardt, J. A., Giovannucci, E. L., Holmes, M. D., Chan, A. T., Chan, J. A., Colditz, G. A., & Fuchs, C. S. (2006). Physical activity and survival after colorectal cancer diagnosis. *Journal of Clinical Oncology, 24*(22), 3527–3534.

Mullens, A. B., McCaul, K. D., Erickson, S. C., & Sandgren, A. K. (2004). Coping after cancer: Risk perceptions, worry, and health behaviors among colorectal cancer survivors. *Psycho-Oncology, 13*(6), 367–376.

Naus, M. J., Price, E. C., & Peter, M. P. (2005). The moderating effects of anxiety and breast cancer locus of control on depression. *Journal of Health Psychology, 10*(5), 687–694.

Rotter, J. B. (1966). Generalized expectancies for internal versus external control of reinforcement. *Psychological Monographs: General and Applied, 80*(1), 1–28.

Schmitz, K. H., Holtzman, J., Courneya, K. S., Mâsse, L. C., Duval, S., & Kane, R. (2005). Controlled physical activity trials in cancer survivors: A systematic review and meta-analysis. *Cancer Epidemiology, Biomarkers and Prevention, 14*(7), 1588–1595.

Schwartz, A. L. (2004). Physical activity after a cancer diagnosis: Psychosocial outcomes. *Cancer Investigation, 22*(1), 82–92.

Siegel, R., DeSantis, C., Virgo, K., Stein, K., Mariotto, A., Smith, T., & Fedewa, S. (2012). Cancer treatment and survivorship statistics, 2012. *CA: A Cancer Journal for Clinicians, 62*(4), 220–241.

Simard, S., & Savard, J. (2009). Fear of cancer recurrence inventory: Development and initial validation of a multidimensional measure of fear of cancer recurrence. *Supportive Care in Cancer, 17*(3), 241–251.

Skaali, T., Fosså, S. D., Bremnes, R., Dahl, O., Haaland, C. F., Hauge, E. R., & Dahl, A. A. (2009). Fear of recurrence in long-term testicular cancer survivors. *Psycho-Oncology, 18*(6), 580–588.

Stanton, A. L., Danoff-burg, S., & Huggins, M. E. (2002). The first year after breast cancer diagnosis: Hope and coping strategies as predictors of adjustment. *Psycho-Oncology, 11*(2), 93–102.

Stanton, A. L., & Reed, G. M. (2003). Coping with treatment side effects. *The breast cancer notebook: The healing power of reflection* (pp. 79–96). Washington, DC, US: American Psychological Association.

Stefanek, M. E., Shaw, A., DeGeorge, D., & Tsottles, N. (1989). Illness-related worry among cancer patients: Prevalence, severity, and content. *Cancer Investigation, 7*(4), 365–371.

Taylor, S. E. (1983). Adjustment to threatening events. *American Psychologist, 38*(11), 1161–1173.

Taylor, S. E., & Brown, J. D. (1994). Positive illusions and well-being revisited: Separating fact from fiction. *Psychological Bulletin, 116*, 21.

Thompson, S. C., & Spacapan, S. (1991). Perceptions of control in vulnerable populations. *Journal of Social Issues, 47*(4), 1–21.

Tran, T. V., Fitzpatrick, T. R., Berg, W. R., & Wright, R, Jr. (1996). Acculturation, health, stress, and psychological distress among elderly Hispanics. *Journal of Cross-Cultural Gerontology, 11*(2), 149–165.

Vickberg, S. M. J. (2003). The concerns about recurrence scale (CARS): A systematic measure of women's fears about the possibility of breast cancer recurrence. *Annals of Behavioral Medicine, 25*(1), 16–24.

Wagner, E. H., LaCroix, A. Z., Buchner, D. M., & Larson, E. B. (1992). Effects of physical activity on health status in older adults I: Observational studies. *Annual Review of Public Health, 13*(1), 451–468.

Watson, M., Pruyn, J., Greek, S., & Van den Borne, B. (1990). Locus of control and adjustment to cancer. *Psychological Reports, 66*(1), 39–48.

Welch-McCaffrey, D., Hoffman, B., Leigh, S. A., Loescher, L. J., & Meyskens, F. L. (1989). Surviving adult cancers. Part 2: Psychosocial implications. *Annals of Internal Medicine, 111* (6), 517–524.

Wheaton, B. (1985). Models for the stress-buffering functions of coping resources. *Journal of Health and Social Behavior*, 352–364.

Young, K. E., & White, C. A. (2006). The prevalence and moderators of fatigue in people who have been successfully treated for cancer. *Journal of Psychosomatic Research, 60*(1), 29–38.

Chapter 8
Oral Health Issues and Quality of Life Among Pediatric Cancer Survivors

Crystal Noronha and Mary Ellen Macdonald

Introduction

Childhood cancer, though relatively rare, is still the second leading cause of death in children under the age of 14 in North America ("Cancer in Children in Canada (0–14 years)," 2012) Whereas twenty years ago, 21 % of children with cancer were surviving each year in North America, aggressive cancer treatment has led to increased survival rates of 83 % in 2014. ("Cancer in Children in Canada (0–14 years)" 2012; Howlader et al. 2014).[1] Many of these curative cancer treatments, however, have serious side-effects for these children, including some which can follow the pediatric cancer survivor long into remission. Importantly, many of these side-effects can affect the oral cavity of the child. Oral side effects can be quite debilitating (Jensen et al. 2010). They can accompany treatment, or show up months—or years—after the initial cancer care (Bagattoni et al. 2014).

Surprisingly, dental care remains a neglected area of pediatric cancer care (da Fonseca 2004; Effinger et al. 2014a, b). The treatment of a child with cancer must involve both curative care alongside the palliative management of any complications resulting from the treatment (Greer et al. 2013). Any area of symptom neglect will ultimately lead to a reduced quality of life (QOL) for the child; oral side-effects are no exception.

[1]The survival rate is the percentage of people in a study or treatment group who are alive five years after their diagnosis or the start of treatment ("Long-Term Follow-Up Guidelines for Survivors of Childhood, Adolescent, and Young Adult Cancers" 2004).

C. Noronha (✉) · M.E. Macdonald
Faculty of Dentistry, McGill University, 2001 McGill College Avenue, Suite 500, Montreal, QC H3A 1G1, Canada
e-mail: crystal.noronha@mcgill.ca

M.E. Macdonald
e-mail: mary.macdonald@mcgill.ca

T.R. Fitzpatrick (ed.), *Treating Vulnerable Populations of Cancer Survivors: A Biopsychosocial Approach*, DOI 10.1007/978-3-319-32364-0_8

This chapter focuses on the oral complications that can follow a pediatric cancer survivor into remission, looking especially at the impact of these side effects on the survivors' QOL. This chapter is based on a scoping review study (Noronha 2012). The goal of this chapter is to describe the types of childhood cancers, the oral side effects that follow their treatment and discuss the implications of these oral effects for the QOL of the pediatric cancer survivors. Suggestions for clinical practice, therapeutic interventions and future research are discussed.

Literature Review

Cancer Survivorship, Quality of Life, and Oral Health

According to the National Cancer Institute (NCI Dictionary of Cancer Terms 2014), the concept of cancer survivorship encompasses "the physical, psychosocial, and economic issues of cancer, from diagnosis until the end of life (http://www.cancer.gov/publications/dictionaries/cancer-terms? (CdrID = 445,089)". This construct of cancer survivorship looks beyond the diagnosis and treatment to also include what occurs after the primary treatment has been completed. For example, after their cancer is treated, many children live with the iatrogenic effects of that treatment—which can include secondary cancers—and lead to reduced QOL.

Quality of Life (QOL) is a broad, multidimensional concept capturing subjective evaluations of positive and negative aspects of life that go beyond clinical status. QOL is defined as the patient's appraisal and satisfaction with their current level of functioning compared to what is perceived to be possible or ideal. QOL can be measured in several domains (e.g., physical, psychological and social) using instruments evaluating the functioning of the patient and the effect on their health condition and on well-being ("Measuring Quality of Life. Retrieved" 1997). The physical aspect encompasses domains such as pain, sleep and rest; psychological aspects are concerned with domains such as body image, feelings, thinking and learning. The social domain includes personal relationships, emotional well-being and social support ("Measuring Quality of Life. Retrieved" 1997).

Quality of life studies are conducted to identify specific problems in psychosocial functioning of the patient and can investigate the secondary effect of treatment regimens on the patient (Fallowfield 2002). In the realm of oncology, studies can make myriad contributions to the understanding of patient experience and the development of patient care interventions. For example, many QOL studies provide comparison of alternate therapies to conventional therapies (Cassileth and Deng 2004), prognostic evaluation of QOL factors (Bradlyn et al. 1996), and can help in identifying late effects of cancer therapy (Bradlyn et al. 1996). Further, these studies can advance decision-making for family members, for example, by providing the financial impact of treatment (Medway et al. 2015).

Quality of life can be assessed in multiple ways. For example, it can be assessed by the patient, by their caregivers and/or by clinicians. Thus, care must be taken when comparing study results. Further, while a patient may often be the best judge of his or her own QOL, patients may report their QOL as being better than it actually is to avoid being troublesome to caregivers. In addition, children and adolescents may not express their feelings and emotions as readily as their parents. Another issue is that clinicians may not have the tools to interpret QOL results.

Effects of Cancer Therapy and Quality of Life for Children

The frequency and intensity of oral side effects and the overall impact on QOL depends on the age of the child during treatment, the intensity of the initial treatment, the stage of tooth development and the location of the cancer. For example, children exposed to radiation treatment before the age of 5 exhibit greater dental effects of treatment than those exposed at later ages (Marec-Berard et al. 2005). Dental caries are an exception, however; they increase in adolescents if the child was treated between the ages of 5 and 6 (Wogelius et al. 2008).

In addition to causing immediate pain and discomfort in the child, the long-term impact of oral complications on the child's oral health is important for many reasons. Children's dentition is constantly developing until adolescence. Neglected oral care during treatment can have an effect on the child both immediately as well as into survivorship. Maintaining good oral health ensures reduction in incidence of dental caries and gum disease, both of which can lead to tooth loss. Both missing teeth and tooth decay are associated with pain, discomfort and problems with eating and sleeping ("Surgeon General's Report on Oral Health" 2014). Tooth loss can also lead to physical, functional, social, emotional and psychological impediments, for example impeding social interaction, communication and basic functions such as chewing and enjoying food. Changes in oral health can also affect voice quality (Mackie et al. 2000). Adolescent cancer survivors especially need psychosocial support as they face psychological distress. A cancer diagnosis coupled with oral health issues affects school life and can isolate the child from their friends (Zebrack et al. 2014). Advances in cancer survivorship rates mean that it is imperative to understand and manage these oral complications to ensure better long-term oral health and QOL for these children.

Childhood Cancers

Childhood cancers differ from adult cancers in type and treatment. Adult cancers are frequently linked to environmental and lifestyle factors; common adult cancers are of the glands or tissues lining organs ("Cancer in Children" 2015). Childhood cancers occur often as a result of changes in cells even before birth and are more commonly blood-related ("Cancer in Children" 2015). Childhood cancers are treated with aggressive treatment regimens, responding better to treatments such as chemotherapy than many adult cancers. The result is that childhood cancers have a better 5-year survival rate than adult cancers (Boklan 2006). The side-effects may be greater, however; both initial and long-term effects of cancer therapy are seen more often in children than in adults since children are at a developing stage; childhood cancer and its treatment are more likely to affect organs that are developing (Pediatric Supportive Care 2015).

Leukemias are the most common types of childhood cancer, occurring in 26 % of cases (Ward et al. 2014). Leukemias arise in the bone marrow and tissues that produce blood cells. Acute lymphoblastic leukemia (ALL) and acute myelogenous leukemia (AML) are the most common. Brain and central nervous system tumors are the second most common type of childhood cancer, occurring in 21 % of cases (Ward et al. 2014). Gliomas, the generic name for tumors that start in the cells of the central nervous system, are the most common type of brain cancer (von Deimling 2009). Lymphomas make up one-fourth of cases in adolescents (Howlader et al. 2014). They arise in the lymph tissue in the body's immune system. Two major types are Hodgkin's lymphoma and non-Hodgkin's lymphoma (Siegel et al. 2015).

Sarcomas are tumors occurring in bones and soft tissue, such as muscles. Osteosarcomas are common types of bone cancers, accounting for 2–3 % of all childhood cancers. Rhabdomyosarcoma, a soft-tissue sarcoma found in the muscles of the head, neck, arms and legs, are the most common soft-tissue sarcomas in children (Ognjanovic et al. 2009). Hepatoblastoma is the most frequently occurring type of liver cancer in children, accounting for just over 1 % of pediatric cancers (Herzog et al. 2000).

Cancers that form in the tissue of the kidneys include Wilm's tumor and clear-cell sarcoma; they are both relatively rare. Other rare childhood cancers include retinoblastoma—a cancer of the retina—and germ cell tumors, which can arise in the testes, ovaries, at the bottom of the spine, as well as in the chest, abdomen and middle of the brain.

Pediatric Cancer Treatment and Its Effect on a Child's Oral Health

Pediatric cancers are treated with chemotherapy, radiotherapy and/or stem cell transplantation. Each of these modalities causes serious side effects, including those that impact the oral cavity of the child. Oral effects occurring during or soon after treatment are classified as early effects; those which occur months later during remission are called late effects (Effinger et al. 2014a, b).

Early Oral Effects

Early oral effects of cancer treatment include xerostomia (dry mouth), oral mucositis, and infections in the mouth and taste disturbances. These side effects range from mild to severe discomfort, and include physical as well as psychosocial distress.

Xerostomia is a subjective feeling of mouth dryness and may be experienced at the early stage of cancer treatment as well as far into remission. It is caused by damage to the salivary glands due to radiation therapy or chemotherapy. Taste disturbances are also similarly caused by radiation therapy or chemotherapy. Both xerostomia and taste disturbances can make all foods taste the same and can make food taste metallic. These effects can lead to food aversions, loss of appetite and weight loss.

Other side effects cause greater physical suffering. Oral mucositis, an acute inflammation and ulceration of the membranes lining the mouth, occurs as a consequence of radiation treatment (either near the mouth or total body irradiation) or high-dose chemotherapy. The pain of oral mucositis can impede a child's ability to eat and drink, thereby reducing nutritional intake and leading to dehydration. Dehydration can in turn increase the risk for xerostomia as well as dental caries; lower nutritional intake can inhibit the body's ability to fight infection and can impede overall recovery. These scenarios can be compounded by radiation injuries to the salivary glands which can affect changes in taste (Otmani 2007; Sonis and Fey 2002).

Importantly, some side-effects can have an immediate effect on the child's treatment regimen. Dental infections, for example, can occur as a result of hematopoietic stem cell transplantation (HSCT) leading to widespread infections in the body. HSCT is a mode of treatment—subsequent to chemotherapy—in which a patient receives bone marrow cells from a donor; it is one of the most severe cancer therapies. Resultant infections can reduce the body's ability to cope with cancer treatment and require treatment interruption until the infection is resolved. Delaying therapy can obviously affect overall treatment outcomes. HSCT therapy can also lead to pain in the mouth, food sensitivities, taste alteration, dryness in the mouth, and restricted movement of the tongue or mouth. Such changes in turn will affect the nutritional status of the child and lowered levels of nutrition can lead to slower recovery ("Guideline on Dental Management of Pediatric Patients Receiving Chemotherapy, Hematopoietic Cell Transplantation, and/or Radiation" 2013).

Late Oral Effects and Quality of Life

The late oral effects of cancer treatment include abnormalities in dental development and jaw development, as well as the development of caries and even secondary tumors at the irradiated sites. These effects can impact current—and delay future—tooth development, with serious physical and psychosocial consequences for the child. As mentioned above, children's dentition is constantly developing until adolescence; so, while the child treated for cancer at a young age may be cured of the cancer, they then can manifest dental abnormalities many years later during remission.

Developmental abnormalities caused by chemotherapy and radiation therapy can result in interrupting the growth of the root; this is called "root stunting." Other common effects of both chemotherapy and radiation therapy include microdontia (a condition of abnormally small teeth), hypodontia (the partial absence of teeth), and the over-retention of primary teeth (Kaste et al. 2009; Minicucci et al. 2003). These long-term effects on dental development may require orthodontic treatment as the child grows (Akharzouz et al. 2013).

Trismus is a side-effect specific to radiation therapy to the jaw, mouth or face. Trismus is the inability to open the jaw wide; this thereby affects a child's speech and ability to eat. It is especially common in patients with nasopharyngeal carcinoma treated with radiation therapy (Özyar et al. 2005).

The risk of developing dental caries (dental decay) is also greatly increased by the effects of some cancer therapies ("Oral complications of cancer therapies: diagnosis, prevention, and treatment" 1989). Dental caries are actually the most common late effect; they are characterized by pits on the tooth surface ("Dental Caries (Tooth Decay)" 2015) and occur when there is change in the quantity of saliva. Damage to the salivary glands by radiotherapy and chemotherapy results in reduced salivary flow, which causes changes in the mouth's environment and increases the chances of developing caries (Gawade et al. 2014).

One parent's experience with the long-term oral effects of cancer treatment and is effect on the QOL of her child:

> A mother of a child in remission for leukemia for four years recounted her child's experience with long-term dental effects of cancer treatment. Her son had a number of cavities and very small teeth. Eating had become an issue and still continued to be a problem. She had never been told about the side-effects of cancer therapy on the mouth and teeth.

As with early effects, many of the late effects co-occur. This can have serious repercussions for the QOL of the child as well as the family. For example, the physical pain that a child may feel in their mouth from the cancer, from the cancer treatment, and/or from the side effects of the treatment, in conjunction with damage, for example, from radiation injuries to the salivary glands thereby affecting salivary production, may seriously affect eating, drinking, and swallowing. Further, the corrective orthodontic procedures and regular follow-up care (Carrillo et al. 2010; Landier et al. 2004), which can follow can entail a large time and financial burden for families.

Methodology

The Scoping Review

A scoping review study was conducted (Noronha 2012) on the relation between oral complications and QOL secondary to treatment in pediatric cancer patients. The scoping review methodology is a type of structured exploratory research review that summarizes and translates existing knowledge for important end-users (e.g., clinicians and researchers) (Grimshaw 2010). In clinical areas where the extent of the research evidence is uncharted—as is the case for oral health in pediatric oncology—a scoping review is an appropriate review methodology because it allows for an in-depth, systematic understanding of an uncharted research field as well as uncovers gaps that require further research. A scoping review differs from a systematic review in that it adopts a broader research question and does not require quality appraisal (Levac et al. 2010).

The goal of this scoping review was exploratory in nature, designed to answer the question: In pediatric oncology patients undergoing therapy (i.e., chemotherapy, radiotherapy, or hematopoietic stem cell transplantation), how do oral complications of the therapy impact the patients' QOL? Our inclusion criteria included the following: articles had to focus on primary research conducted between 2000 and 2011, be published in English or French, and focus on children (0–20 years old) with any type of cancer who had undergone chemotherapy, radiotherapy or HSCT and who exhibited early or late oral effect of cancer therapy. The databases from which we sought published articles included Medline, Embase, CINAHL, Global Health, The Allied and Complementary Medicine Database (AMED), PsycINFO, Cochrane Library, Database of Abstracts of Reviews of (DARE) and Proquest Dissertations and Theses. Unpublished studies were identified through the following databases: ISI Web of Science, Scopus, Open Grey, New York Academy of Medicine (NYAM), WorldCat and through websites of dental and oncology organizations such as the International Association for Dental Research and International Society of Pediatric Oncology (see Appendix 1 for the resultant literature search process; the extensive results of this review can be found in Noronha 2012).

Findings

Management of Quality of Life Issues

As described earlier, activities of daily living such as eating, talking, smiling, and personal mouth care are affected by a child's cancer therapy. For those clinicians working with caregivers, it is important to help them understand the kinds of food that the child can manage in order to ensure both adequate nutrition as well as some pleasure when eating. If the child is assisted in choosing foods that are manageable given his or her oral condition, this can improve nutrition. Cheng (2009) found that maintaining personal mouth care was an issue for children with cancer; they felt pressure from parents to maintain oral hygiene. In the words of one child, "*Yes, my Dad forced me to do it. Mum also forced me to do it*" (Cheng 2009). Children considered mouth care a forced activity despite the discomfort caused by the pain involved. Further, the unpleasant taste of mouthwash was an issue.

Psychological and Social Domains

The psychological and social domains of a child's QOL overlap in important ways. For example, Cheng (2009) evaluated the effect of oral mucositis on pediatric cancer patients and found it to have both psychological and social impacts. Additionally, speech issues associated with oral mucositis can contribute to the adolescent patient's reluctance to engage in social interaction.

Similarly, Green et al. (2010) documented the impact on various dimensions of QOL through patient interviews (Green et al. 2010). The following verbatim speaks about the importance of the issue of oral complications such as mucositis: *When people talked to me, I couldn't answer them, and they'd think that I was ignoring them. I had an oral ulcer and I couldn't speak. I wanted to talk but I couldn't. People didn't know that. My friends found it strange that I became so introverted* (informant 2—child) (Cheng 2009). Children in Green's study described mouth soreness as making eating hard and painful; however, they developed their own strategies to combat mouth problems such as taking pain medication before eating, eating foods like toast that were tolerated and experimenting with foods (Green et al. 2010).

Many cancer treatments, such as treatment for brain tumors, result in absences from school and learning problems (Upton and Eiser 2006). On the other hand, for adolescents, a return to school can signify a transition to a new life. Cancer treatment encompassing management of psychosocial issues is an important area that should be further developed (Choquette et al. 2015).

Physical Domain

The physical domain includes pain, sleep and rest. The physical pain that the patient feels in their mouth affects their ability to eat and contributes to changes in taste. Thus, eating, drinking, and swallowing are affected. These changes affect the child's nutritional status (Bauer et al. 2011). Control of pain can aid in better management of nutritional issues.

Multi-disciplinary Approach in Pediatric Cancer Care

The findings from this scoping review highlight the need for health care professionals treating pediatric cancer patients to be aware of the necessity of a team approach that includes a pediatric dentist. Oral care for pediatric cancer survivors should begin before cancer treatment commences. Referral to a pediatric dentist prior to treatment and constant monitoring of oral health issues during cancer treatment can lead to better dental—and overall—health outcomes. As oral complications of cancer therapy have an effect on the QOL of the pediatric cancer patient, there is a need for inter-professional collaboration among the related health fields such as dentistry, pediatric oncology, nursing and the allied health fields.

The increase in survival rates of childhood cancer necessitates the integration of a preventive oral care protocol in pediatric oncology treatment to reduce oral effects of cancer treatment in cancer survivors. Treatment and follow-up care of pediatric cancer patients requires a multi-disciplinary approach. The intensity of the oral complications depends on the site of the cancer, the intensity of the treatment, the age of the child, the status of oral and dental health, and the level of dental care before, during, and after therapy. Adequate and timely oral care minimizes the risk of oral complications during cancer therapy and through cancer survivorship. Therapy-related oral complications may not get entirely eliminated; however, they can be minimized and preventive oral care can aid in re-focusing attention onto the cancer treatment.

There are inconsistencies in mouth care in hospitals from the perspective of nursing staff due to lack of guidelines and education (Glenny et al. 2004). Nurses often lack adequate knowledge about mouth care leading to this task not being routinely carried out (Glenny et al. 2004). Increased education on mouth care and coordination with the hospital dentist would assist nurses in giving adequate mouth care to children. Implementation of oral care guidelines such as those developed by the National Institute of Dental and Craniofacial Research ("Oral Complications of Cancer Treatment: What the Dental Team Can Do" 2014) can help nurses and patients to maintain standards of oral hygiene.

Adequate and timely oral care of pediatric cancer patients minimizes the risk of oral complications during cancer therapy. Work by Glenny (2004), and colleagues underscores the importance of dental care during cancer treatment (Glenny et al. 2004) reporting that only 36 % of cancer centers in the United Kingdom sent pediatric cancer patients for oral checkups before the cancer treatment (Glenny et al. 2004). Therapy-related oral complications may not get entirely addressed, however, they can be minimized and preventive oral care can aid in focusing attention on cancer treatment. The oral cavity is a part of the body and needs to be treated in conjunction with the rest of the body to minimize effects on general health.

Discussion

This chapter summarizes the results of our scoping review, specifically focusing on how the oral complications of cancer therapy compromise QOL for pediatric cancer survivors. The findings from these studies confirm that pediatric cancer survivors face several QOL issues related to oral health and cancer treatment. Pain is a common factor throughout these studies. If mouth pain can be controlled, it can lead to a better QOL for the child.

Cancer treatment effects have a functional, social, emotional and psychological impact. It is important to measure QOL especially in the adolescent patient as the teenage years represent physical and psychological development of the individual such as personal relationships, sexuality, employment, and financial issues. There are challenges in providing care to this population. Cancer treatment disrupts several areas of the adolescents' life not only with an invasive treatment but also in areas such as education, peer relations, emotions, body image and self-esteem (Nass et al. 2015). Psychosocial support and palliative care are also important components of cancer care. Long-term follow-up care should include both physical and psychological screening as pediatric cancer survivors face difficulties reestablishing their lives at the school, home, and community level (Aldridge and Roesch 2007).

There is a growing body of international research on the oral complications faced by pediatric cancer survivors subsequent to cancer therapy, yet, few use qualitative methods. Using qualitative methods can enhance our understanding of the psychosocial issues faced by this vulnerable population (Tonon 2015). There are also few studies from Canada, which show the potential for further research in this area (Bakish et al. 2003; Manji et al. 2012).

Our study suggests that caregivers need to be educated on mouth care for pediatric cancer patients. Education could involve increased training for allied health care staff as well as for parents and families. Preventive care can lead to uninterrupted cancer treatment, better outcomes, and a better QOL for the pediatric cancer survivor.

Areas for Future Research

There is a lack of longitudinal studies evaluating the effect of psychosocial interventions and their impact on a pediatric cancer survivor's oral health in the long term. Longitudinal studies and clinical trials of early oral effects can demonstrate the impact of these complications and aid treatment decision-making (Efficace et al. 2014). Most studies focus on oral mucositis and not on the other oral complications that affect a pediatric cancer survivor undergoing cancer treatment (Noronha 2012). There is relatively little attention paid to the impact of oral complications on QOL of the pediatric cancer survivor, especially using qualitative methods. Our study showed that using qualitative methods can provide further insight into the psychosocial issues faced by the cancer patient, which may not easily be drawn from clinical trials (Rodgers et al. 2010). Proxy ratings of QOL may be used in a child too ill to give his/her own evaluation of QOL. When assessing QOL related to oral health, the whole person and not just the mouth has to be considered necessitating psychosocial interventions. Oral health is a window to general health and the mouth is not a separate entity from the rest of the body.

Conclusions

An increase in survival rates of childhood cancer necessitates the integration of a preventive oral care protocol in pediatric oncology treatment to reduce oral effects of cancer treatment. It is clear that oral complications of cancer therapy have an effect on the QOL of the pediatric cancer survivor. This chapter demonstrates the need for an inter-professional collaboration in the treatment of pediatric cancer and the need for the inclusion of a dentist on the pediatric oncology team to provide preventive oral care. Children's dentition is constantly developing into adolescence and neglected oral care during treatment can have an effect on the child in remission and survivorship. Understanding that QOL is affected by cancer treatment-related oral complications may help health care professionals give more comprehensive care and attention to their patients and the issues family members experience. The treatment focus must be on the cancer; however, mitigating the side-effects of the treatment can lead to an improvement in the pediatric cancer survivors' QOL.

Acknowledgements I would like to thank Dr. Mary Ellen Macdonald and Dr. Tanya Fitzpatrick for their invaluable support in editing this chapter. I would also like to thank Dr. Christophe Bedos, the members of the Oral Health, and Society research unit and the members of the Pediatric Palliative Care Research Rounds at the Montreal Children's Hospital for their advice during the initial study.

Appendix 1: PRISMA Flow Diagram

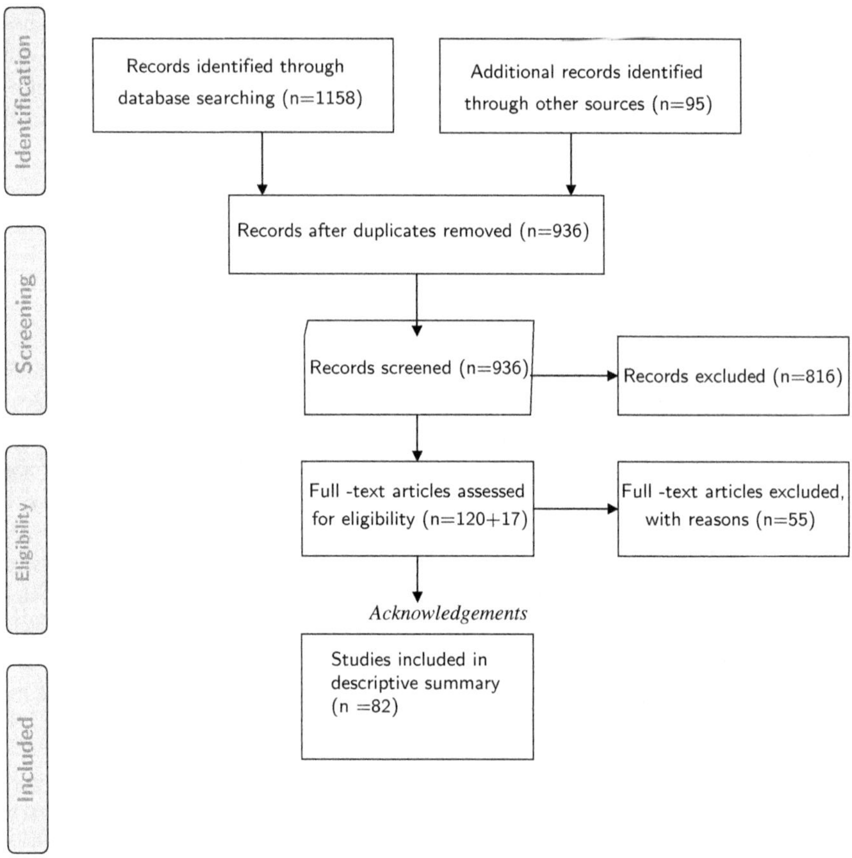

References

Akharzouz, C., Chauty, S., & Bodard, A. G. (2013). Children who received a radiotherapy treatment of the cranio-cervico-facial region: Appraisal of the orthodontic treatment need. *Orthodontie Francaise, 84*(2), 157–168. doi:10.1051/orthodfr/2013047

Aldridge, A., & Roesch, S. (2007). Coping and adjustment in children with cancer: A meta-analytic study. *Journal of Behavioral Medicine, 30*(2), 115–129. doi:10.1007/s10865-006-9087-y

Bagattoni, S., D'Alessandro, G., Prete, A., Piana, G., & Pession, A. (2014). Oral health and dental late adverse effects in children in remission from malignant disease. A pilot case-control study in Italian children. *European Journal of Paediatric Dentistry, 15*(1), 45–50.

Bakish, J., Hargrave, D., Tariq, N., Laperriere, N., Rutka, J. T., & Bouffet, E. (2003). Evaluation of dietetic intervention in children with medulloblastoma or supratentorial primitive neuroectodermal tumors. *Cancer, 98*(5), 1014–1020. doi:10.1002/cncr.11598

Bauer, J., Jürgens, H., & Frühwald, M. C. (2011). Important aspects of nutrition in children with cancer. *Advances in Nutrition: An International Review Journal, 2*(2), 67–77. doi:10.3945/an.110.000141

Boklan, J. (2006). Little patients, losing patience: Pediatric cancer drug development. *Molecular Cancer Therapeutics, 5*(8), 1905–1908. doi:10.1158/1535-7163.mct-06-0179

Bradlyn, A. S., Ritchey, A. K., Harris, C. V., Moore, I. M., O'Brien, R. T., Parsons, S. K., & Pollock, B. H. (1996). Quality of life research in pediatric oncology: Research methods and barriers. *Cancer, 78*(6), 1333–1339. doi:10.1002/(sici)1097-0142(19960915)78:6<1333:aid-cncr24>3.0.co;2-0

Cancer in Children. (2015, January 13, 2015) Retrieved October 15, 2015, from http://www.cancer.org/cancer/cancerinchildren/detailedguide/cancer-in-children-differences-adults-children

Cancer in Children in Canada (0–14 years). (2012, July 09) Retrieved May 30, 2015, from http://www.phac-aspc.gc.ca/cd-mc/cancer/fs-fi/cancer-child-enfant/index-eng.php#sur

Carrillo, C., Vizeu, H., Soares-Júnior, L. A., Fava, M., & Filho, V. O. (2010). Dental approach in the pediatric oncology patient: Characteristics of the population treated at the dentistry unit in a pediatric oncology Brazilian teaching hospital. *Clinics, 65*(6), 569–573. doi:10.1590/s1807-59322010000600002

Cassileth, B. R., & Deng, G. (2004). Complementary and alternative therapies for cancer. *The Oncologist, 9*(1), 80–89. doi:10.1634/theoncologist.9-1-80

Cheng, K. K. (2009). Oral mucositis: A phenomenological study of pediatric patients' and their parents' perspectives and experiences. *Supportive Care in Cancer, 17*(7), 829–837. doi:10.1007/s00520-009-0618-2

Choquette, A., Rennick, J. E., & Lee, V. (2015). Back to school after cancer treatment: Making sense of the adolescent experience. *Cancer Nursing,*. doi:10.1097/ncc.0000000000000301

da Fonseca, M. A. (2004). Dental care of the pediatric cancer patient. *Pediatric Dentistry, 26*(1), 53–57.

Dental Caries (Tooth Decay). (2015) Retrieved Oct 18, 2015.

Efficace, F., Jacobs, M., Pusic, A., Greimel, E., Piciocchi, A., Kieffer, J. M., & Blazeby, J. (2014). Patient-reported outcomes in randomised controlled trials of gynaecological cancers: Investigating methodological quality and impact on clinical decision-making. *European Journal of Cancer, 50*(11), 1925–1941. doi:10.1016/j.ejca.2014.04.005

Effinger, K., Migliorati, C., Hudson, M., McMullen, K., Kaste, S., Ruble, K., & Castellino, S. (2014a). Oral and dental late effects in survivors of childhood cancer: A children's oncology group report. *Supportive Care in Cancer, 22*(7), 2009–2019. doi:10.1007/s00520-014-2260-x

Effinger, K. E., Migliorati, C. A., Hudson, M. M., McMullen, K. P., Kaste, S. C., Ruble, K., & Castellino, S. M. (2014b). Oral and dental late effects in survivors of childhood cancer: A children's oncology group report. *Supportive Care in Cancer, 22*(7), 2009–2019. doi:10.1007/s00520-014-2260-x

Fallowfield, L. (2002). Quality of life: A new perspective for cancer patients. *Nature Reviews Cancer, 2*(11), 873–879. doi:10.1038/nrc930

Gawade, P. L., Hudson, M. M., Kaste, S. C., Neglia, J. P., Constine, L. S., Robison, L. L., & Ness, K. K. (2014). A systematic review of dental late effects in survivors of childhood cancer. *Pediatric Blood & Cancer, 61*(3), 407–416. doi:10.1002/pbc.24842

Glenny, A. M., Gibson, F., Auld, E., Coulson, S., Clarkson, J. E., Craig, J. V., & Pizer, B. (2004). A survey of current practice with regard to oral care for children being treated for cancer. *European Journal of Cancer, 40*(8), 1217–1224. doi:10.1016/j.ejca.2004.01.030

Green, R., Horn, H., & Erickson, J. M. (2010). Eating experiences of children and adolescents with chemotherapy-related nausea and mucositis. *Journal of Pediatric Oncology Nursing, 27*(4), 209–216. doi:10.1177/1043454209360779

Greer, J. A., Jackson, V. A., Meier, D. E., & Temel, J. S. (2013). Early integration of palliative care services with standard oncology care for patients with advanced cancer. *CA: A Cancer Journal for Clinicians, 63*(5), 349–363. doi:10.3322/caac.21192

Grimshaw, J. (2010, Apr 8). A guide to knowledge synthesis. Retrieved Oct 18, 2015, from http://www.cihr-irsc.gc.ca/e/41382.html

Guideline on dental management of pediatric patients receiving chemotherapy, hematopoietic cell transplantation, and/or radiation. *Pediatric Dentistry, 35*(5), 185E–193E, 2013.

Herzog, C. E., Andrassy, R. J., & Eftekhari, F. (2000). Childhood cancers: Hepatoblastoma. *The Oncologist, 5*(6), 445–453. doi:10.1634/theoncologist.5-6-445

Howlader, N., Noone, A., Krapcho, M., Garshell, J., Miller, D., Altekruse, S., & Cronin, K. (2014, Apr 2015). SEER cancer statistics review. 1975–2012, Nov 2014. Retrieved June 14, 2015, from http://seer.cancer.gov/csr/1975_2012/

Jensen, S. B., Pedersen, A. M., Vissink, A., Andersen, E., Brown, C. G., Davies, A. N., & Brennan, M. T. (2010). A systematic review of salivary gland hypofunction and xerostomia induced by cancer therapies: Prevalence, severity and impact on quality of life. *Supportive Care in Cancer, 18*(8), 1039–1060. doi:10.1007/s00520-010-0827-8

Kaste, S. C., Goodman, P., Leisenring, W., Stovall, M., Hayashi, R., Yeazel, M., & Baker, K. S. (2009). Impact of radiation and chemotherapy on risk of dental abnormalities: A report from the childhood cancer survivor study. *Cancer, 115*(24), 5817–5827. doi:10.1002/cncr.24670

Landier, W., Bhatia, S., Eshelman, D. A., Forte, K. J., Sweeney, T., Hester, A. L., & Hudson, M. M. (2004). Development of risk-based guidelines for pediatric cancer survivors: The children's oncology group long-term follow-up guidelines from the children's oncology group late effects committee and nursing discipline. *Journal of Clinical Oncology, 22*(24), 4979–4990. doi:10.1200/jco.2004.11.032

Levac, D., Colquhoun, H., & O'Brien, K. K. (2010). Scoping studies: Advancing the methodology. *Implementation Science: IS, 5*, 69. doi:10.1186/1748-5908-5-69

Mackie, A. M., Epstein, J. B., Wu, J. S. Y., & Stevenson-Moore, P. (2000). Nasopharyngeal carcinoma: The role of the dentist in assessment, early diagnosis and care before and after cancer therapy. *Oral Oncology, 36*(5), 397–403. doi:10.1016/S1368-8375(00)00034-8

Manji, A., Tomlinson, D., Ethier, M. C., Gassas, A., Maloney, A. M., & Sung, L. (2012). Psychometric properties of the oral mucositis daily questionnaire for child self-report and importance of mucositis in children treated with chemotherapy. *Supportive Care in Cancer, 20*(6), 1251–1258. doi:10.1007/s00520-011-1211-z

Marec-Berard, P., Azzi, D., Chaux-Bodard, A. G., Lagrange, H., Gourmet, R., & Bergeron, C. (2005). Long-term effects of chemotherapy on dental status in children treated for nephroblastoma. *Pediatric Hematology and Oncology, 22*(7), 581–588. doi:10.1080/08880010500198848

Measuring Quality of Life. Retrieved. (1997). Retrieved June 6, 2015, from http://www.who.int/mental_health/media/68.pdf

Medway, M., Tong, A., Craig, J. C., Kim, S., Mackie, F., McTaggart, S., & Wong, G. (2015). Parental perspectives on the financial impact of caring for a child with CKD. *American Journal of Kidney Diseases, 65*(3), 384–393. doi:10.1053/j.ajkd.2014.07.019

Minicucci, E. M., Lopes, L. F., & Crocci, A. J. (2003). Dental abnormalities in children after chemotherapy treatment for acute lymphoid leukemia. *Leukemia Research, 27*(1), 45–50.

Nass, S. J., Beaupin, L. K., Demark-Wahnefried, W., Fasciano, K., Ganz, P. A., Hayes-Lattin, B., & Smith, A. W. (2015). Identifying and addressing the needs of adolescents and young adults with cancer: Summary of an institute of medicine workshop. *Oncologist, 20*(2), 186–195. doi:10.1634/theoncologist.2014-0265

NCI Dictionary of Cancer Terms (2014) National Cancer Institute. Retrieved September/October, 2015, from http://www.cancer.gov/publications/dictionaries/cancer-terms

Noronha, C. (2012). Impact on quality of life due to therapy-related oral complications in pediatric cancer patients: A scoping review. M.Sc. Manuscript based, McGill Univeristy, Montreal, Canada.

Ognjanovic, S., Linabery, A. M., Charbonneau, B., & Ross, J. A. (2009). Trends in childhood rhabdomyosarcoma incidence and survival in the United States (1975–2005). *Cancer, 115*(18), 4218–4226. doi:10.1002/cncr.24465

Oral complications of cancer therapies: Diagnosis, prevention, and treatment. National Institute of Health Consensus Development Conference Consensus Statement, *7*(7), 1–11, 1989.

Oral complications of cancer treatment: what the dental team can do, 2014. Retrieved Oct 18, 2015, from http://www.nidcr.nih.gov/oralhealth/Topics/CancerTreatment/OralComplications CancerOral.htm#5

Otmani, N. (2007). Oral and maxillofacial side effects of radiation therapy on children. *Journal/Canadian Dental Association. Journal de l'Association Dentaire Canadienne, 73*(3), 257–261.

Özyar, E., Cengiz, M., Gurkaynak, M., & Atahan, I. L. (2005). Trismus as a presenting symptom in nasopharyngeal carcinoma. *Radiotherapy and Oncology, 77*(1), 73–76. doi:10.1016/j.radonc.2005.07.006

Pediatric Supportive Care. (2015, Jan 22) Retrieved Oct 15, 2015, from http://www.cancer.gov/types/childhood-cancers/pediatric-care-pdq

Rodgers, C., Young, A., Hockenberry, M., Binder, B., & Symes, L. (2010). The meaning of adolescents' eating experiences during bone marrow transplant recovery. *Journal of Pediatric Oncology Nursing, 27*(2), 65–72. doi:10.1177/1043454209355984

Siegel, R. L., Miller, K. D., & Jemal, A. (2015). Cancer statistics, 2015. *CA: A Cancer Journal for Clinicians, 65*(1), 5–29. doi:10.3322/caac.21254

Sonis, S. T., & Fey, E. G. (2002). Oral complications of cancer therapy. *Oncology (Williston Park), 16*(5), 680–686; discussion 686, 691–682, 695.

Surgeon General's Report on Oral Health. (2014, March 7). Retrieved Oct 13, 2015, from http://www.nidcr.nih.gov/DataStatistics/SurgeonGeneral/

Tonon, G. (2015). *Qualitative studies in quality of life: Methodology and practice*. Springer International Publishing.

Upton, P., & Eiser, C. (2006). School experiences after treatment for a brain tumour. *Child: Care, Health and Development, 32*(1), 9–17. doi:10.1111/j.1365-2214.2006.00569.x

von Deimling, A. (2009). *Gliomas*. Berlin, Heidelberg: Springer.

Ward, E., DeSantis, C., Robbins, A., Kohler, B., & Jemal, A. (2014). Childhood and adolescent cancer statistics, 2014. *CA: A Cancer Journal for Clinicians, 64*(2), 83–103. doi:10.3322/caac.21219

Wogelius, P., Dahllof, G., Gorst-Rasmussen, A., Sorensen, H. T., Rosthoj, S., & Poulsen, S. (2008). A population-based observational study of dental caries among survivors of childhood cancer. *Pediatric Blood & Cancer, 50*(6), 1221–1226. doi:10.1002/pbc.21464

Zebrack, B. J., Corbett, V., Embry, L., Aguilar, C., Meeske, K. A., Hayes-Lattin, B., & Cole, S. (2014). Psychological distress and unsatisfied need for psychosocial support in adolescent and young adult cancer patients during the first year following diagnosis. *Psychooncology, 23*(11), 1267–1275. doi:10.1002/pon.3533

Chapter 9
Quality of Life Among Esophageal Cancer Survivors: Medical and Psychosocial Support

Adriano Petrangelo, Mara L. Leimanis, Lorenzo Ferri and Tanya R. Fitzpatrick

Introduction

Epidemiology and Demographics

Currently the eighth most common malignancy worldwide, an estimated 456,000 people, are diagnosed with esophageal cancer every year (Torre et al. 2015). Annually 17,000 Americans and 2200 Canadians will be diagnosed with this cancer disease, with 16,000 and 2100 people, respectively, dying from the disease (Canadian Cancer Society's Advisory Committee on Cancer Statistics 2015).

A. Petrangelo (✉)
Department of Surgery, McGill University, 8824 Girardin, Montreal, QC H1R 2E5, Canada
e-mail: Adriano.petrangelo@mail.mcgill.ca

M.L. Leimanis
1221 Oxbow Drive, Middleville, MI 49333, USA
e-mail: mara.leimanis@spectrumhealth.org

L. Ferri
Department of Surgery, Montreal General Hospital, McGill University, Room L9-112, 1650 Cedar Avenue, Montreal, QC H3G 1A4, Canada
e-mail: Lorenzo.ferri@mcgill.ca

T.R. Fitzpatrick
Department of Nursing, McGill University, 449 Mount Pleasant Ave, Westmount, QC H3Y3G9, Canada
e-mail: tanya.fitzpatrick@asu.edu

T.R. Fitzpatrick (ed.), *Treating Vulnerable Populations of Cancer Survivors: A Biopsychosocial Approach*, DOI 10.1007/978-3-319-32364-0_9

Key Statistics About Cancer of the Esophagus

Men are seven times more likely to develop this disease compared with women (Rustgi and El-Serag 2014). A disease very uncommon in people under the age of 45 (<2 % of diagnoses) rates peak in the seventh to eighth decades of life (Fact Sheets: Esophageal Cancer 2015). However, esophageal cancer is not a very common cancer in the Western World in comparison to its incidence rates in many developing countries, where the disease is considered to be endemic (Ajani et al. 2011) such as the so-called "esophageal cancer belt" spanning the region from northern Iran to northern China (Patel et al. 2013). However, recent epidemiological data is worrying. Researchers examining data from the United States and the United Kingdom consider the cancer to be on an "epidemic rise" in these areas, with incidence rates having increased fivefold in the past 30 years (Abrams 2009). Furthermore, when compared with 30 years ago, the average male is 50 % more likely to develop esophageal cancer, and this statistic continues to rise (Cancer Research UK 2015).

Risk factors for esophageal cancer include excessive alcohol consumption, tobacco use, gastroesophageal reflux disease, diets poor in fruits and vegetables, and obesity. Experts suggest the surge in incidence seen in the past 30 years can be attributed to the parallel growth of obesity rates seen in the Western World (Alexandre et al. 2014). While it may not be as common as breast, colon or other forms of prevalent cancer diseases, esophageal cancer is a growing concern, validating an increased awareness and education of the disease for workers in the health care field.

Literature Review

Connecting the oral pharynx to the stomach, the esophagus is a muscular tube bridging three anatomical compartments, the neck, thorax and abdomen. It is surrounded on its sides by the two lungs, with the trachea or heart in front, and the spinal column in back. It has an average length of 25 cm (Mescher and Junqueira 2013).

At a cellular level, the esophagus is seen as being composed of three main layers. The outermost layer, or muscularis propria, is composed of muscle cells. This muscle tissue allows the esophagus to contract in a controlled wave and push food towards the stomach, in a process that is known as peristalsis. The middle layer, the submucosa, is composed of vasculature, nerves, lymphatic vessels, and loose connective tissue. The innermost layer, the mucosa, is the layer in contact with the lumen of the esophagus, where the boluses of food will pass on their path to the stomach. As such, the mucosa itself is composed of epithelial cells, protecting it from the abrasive potential of the boluses as well as many mucosal glands, which produce and secrete mucous that allows for a smoother passage of the boluses (Mescher and Junqueira 2013).

In response to environmental injury and stresses, such as those induced by alcohol, cigarette smoke, or refluxed acid and bile from the stomach, cells of the esophagus may start to behave abnormally. Accumulation of injuries from these stressors may induce changes within the esophageal mucosal cells ultimately leading to malignant transformation and the development of esophageal cancer. Depending on the injurious agent the esophageal mucosal cells can develop into either squamous cell carcinoma (in response to smoking and alcohol) or adenocarcinoma (in response to gastroesophageal reflux disease). Although worldwide squamous cell carcinoma is the most common form, in Europe and North America, adenocarcinoma in by far the most prevalent histologic subtype of esophageal cancer. Indeed, the National Cancer Institute has identified adenocarcinoma of the esophagus the fastest growing subtype of cancer in the United States (Talley et al. 2010).

Patients normally present to the clinic with problems swallowing, known as dysphagia, caused by the obstruction of the lumen of the esophagus by the tumor mass. However, due to the expandable nature of the esophagus, partial occlusions of its lumen due to growing malignancies can remain asymptomatic for quite some time. For this reasons, most patients who present to the clinic are already in an advanced stage of the disease (Cools-Lartigue et al. 2015).

Treatment for esophageal cancer is complex and based primarily on both patient and tumor factors (recently reviewed in Cools-Lartigue et al. 2015). Early stage patients (stage I) typically undergo either endoscopic or laparoscopic resection, while patients with more locally advanced disease (stage II–III) often require multimodal therapy (chemotherapy or chemo-radiotherapy prior to an operation). Treatment for those with advanced or unresectable disease centers around palliation of symptoms with either chemotherapy, radiotherapy, or endoscopic treatments. It is important to note that the primary goal of treatment in patients with metastatic esophageal cancer is providing the best quality of life for the longest time possible.

Prognosis for the patient is influenced by many factors, with the most reliable being the stage of the cancer (Cools-Lartigue et al. 2015). As mentioned however, most people present to the clinic with an already advanced stage of disease. Studies have shown 90 % of patients present to the clinic with a late-stage disease, irrespective of the histological subtype (Schlansky et al. 2006). The aggressive nature of this disease, as well as the late stage of presentation, translate into esophageal cancer having one of the worst prognoses of solid organ malignancies, with an overall 5-year survival of approximately 15 % (Canadian Cancer Society's Advisory Committee on Cancer Statistics 2015).

Quality of Life

Cancer diagnoses have a profound impact on the lives of the millions of people diagnosed with the disease every year. Words alone would not do justice to the burden placed upon the patient, their family, and their social group throughout their treatment and recovery. Every person who walks into a cancer treatment center every day comes from a different social background, a different economic background, and a different psychological background. They belong to families, to social groups, to workplaces, or to recreational activities. Each diagnosis brings with it more than just a malignancy and a treatment plan. It brings uncertainty and distress disability, possible financial difficulties, social burdens, and psychological burdens. And for each different patient, the complex web of these problems will be different. Social workers, doctors, nutritionists, nurses, and support staff will need to focus their interventions with a treatment plan unique for each and every survivor. The ultimate goal is to provide appropriate support directed towards improving their quality of life. Words from a surgeon:

> I usually focus on the goal, we treat everyone as individuals, as every person with cancer is different, and we want to aim for the best quality of life for the longest possible time.

Quality of life is a broad multidimensional concept including subjective evaluations of various aspects of a patient's life. While health constitutes a part of one's quality of life, other factors such as economic status, social status, and psychological status also influence one's well-being. For this reason researchers and health practitioners use Health Related Quality of Life, or HRQoL. HRQoL, in short, can be understood as "assessment by the patient of the impact that a medical condition or treatment has on some aspect of their functioning" (DeVita et al. 2008, p. 344). It encompasses measuring physical, psychological, and social function quantitatively. Words from an oncology nurse specialist from a busy esophageal cancer program:

> The initial "triage" for me revolves around the 4 following issues: 1) ECOG, 2) resources: do they have meaningful family relationships, significant others, partners, who can support in the treatment trajectory, and intervene on their behalf, 3) economical: what is their economic reality? As there will be additional expenses, so their economic status plays a part. ex: if they have to spend "x" amount for anti-nausea medications, but can't afford it, this will affect their care, and how I deal with their care. Or, do they have transport? If they can not afford transport, can we arrange it with a social worker, 4) psychosocial: what is their coping history? Do they have a history of mental health issues, as cancer will cause additional stresses. If they have limited coping skills, I will refer to psychosocial oncology. This can vary greatly from the patient commenting "I feel depressed"…I will then explore if they are on medication or not, which is a different conversation than "I feel like I want to end my life."

We must question, however, what is the true importance of attempting to quantify and keep track longitudinally, a patient's HRQoL throughout treatment, specifically in regard to treatment of esophageal cancer. Why not just treat the cancer as aggressively as possible to give the patient the best chance of recovery, regardless of the strains it will place upon them? If two different patients, of similar age and medical history, present with similar stage cancer and similar cancer type, should they both be treated the same regardless of their different longitudinal fluctuations in HRQoL? The answer is complex but also illustrates the beauty of the art of medicine, which goes beyond the scope of basic science and textbooks. When facing a disease such as esophageal cancer that has a high mortality rate, health care professionals must find a balance between cure and maintaining a patient's HRQoL to the best of their abilities, should a cure not be achieved.

It is only in the past decade that we have moved past examining the side effects of medical treatment, effectiveness of treatment in terms of survival and treatment-related mortality and started to recognize HRQoL as a clinically relevant indicator of therapy outcome (Darling 2013). Keeping the patient's HRQoL in mind in all interventions is important as it gives a greater understanding of a patient's status, going beyond what can be seen under a microscope, imaging, and tests. It may seem as too subjective a measure to some, yet multiple studies dealing with patients with esophageal cancer have shown studying the longitudinal progression of a patient's HRQoL is a strong tool for evaluating their prognosis, chances for other morbidities, and mortality (Kypriotakis et al. 2015; Djarv et al. 2008). Furthermore, a study by McNair et al. questioned patients to rank, in order of importance, their information needs when diagnosed with esophageal cancer. Receiving information on the tests they will undergo, their treatment along with the nature, process and prognosis of their cancer were all deemed of importance to them, but they ranked physical and psychosocial outcomes, or their HRQoL, as the most important information need (McNair et al. 2013).

Quantifying and following a patient's HRQoL longitudinally is not without its challenges as a clinically relevant measure. Even though we have studied, and continue to study, its importance during cancer treatment, a unified standard system to measure HRQoL has not been instituted. There are multiple different HRQoL questionnaires being used by researchers and health care professionals, creating problems for quantitatively interpreting HRQoL scores across the different formats (Trask et al. 2009). Each of these different questionnaires also may ask the patient different questions, in a different way, making comparison of these scores even more subjective. The current recommendation is to use either the European Organization for the Research and Treatment of Cancer (EORTC), Quality of Life Questionnaire-Core 30 (QLQ-C30), or the Functional Assessment of Cancer Therapy (FACT), which have proven their validity in many clinical trials (Trask et al. 2009). Burden placed on the patient to complete the survey should also be considered. Depending on their trajectory of treatment, state of mind, prognosis and interest, patients may sometimes feel taxed in completing long surveys about many aspects of their mental and physical health state. It may unduly exacerbate their anxiety about their condition, especially if they feel completing the survey will have little to no impact on their own treatment outlook, which should be monitored by qualified clinical staff such a social worker who may be able to triage their immediate needs and concerns, such as pain (Trask et al. 2009). Finally, a cancer center having the logistical resources to administer these questionnaires to survivors with their every visit and then take the time to record and interpret the results may be out of the question for most centers (Trask et al. 2009).

These challenges are all understandable and it may be unreasonable to believe cancer centers across the world will adopt administering and interpreting HRQoL questionnaires overnight. The good news is, nurses, social workers, nutritionists, psychosocial oncologists, doctors and support staff can, and should, simply take into consideration a patient's HRQoL during their treatment in whichever way they deem fit.

The following section will delve into the separate modalities of therapeutic interventions for patients with esophageal cancer, by first assessing the challenges faced as it pertains to their HRQoL and second by summarizing how health care workers address these issues.

Therapeutic Interventions

Social Support as a Concept

Social support is a multimodal concept aiming to describe the perception that one is being cared for by their social network. Gottlieb and Bengen (2009) define social support as "The social resources that persons perceive to be available or that are actually provided to them by nonprofessionals in the context of both formal support groups and informal helping relationships" (2009, p. 511). While humans possess biological imperatives such as self-preservation and reproduction as seemingly every other species on earth, we are without a doubt the most social. Darwin himself theorized the human race's survival was "contingent on people's ability to 'sympathetically' co-exist with each other" (Rab 2012, p. 31). Humans' propensity to form meaningful relationships and develop interpersonal dependence remains unmatched in the animal kingdom.

The relationships formed within our network do provide us with the astonishing ability to provide social support to other members of our species, but also leave us vulnerable as our social nature forces us to be dependent upon those with whom we have public and social ties. Studies have shown a strong interconnectedness between one's health and well-being and the health and well-being of others in their social network. For example, studies have linked declining physical health in one spouse to declining health in the spousal caregiver, likely due to the high levels of stress placed upon them (Schulz and Beach 1999). On the other hand, increased social support has been shown to increase the subjective well-being of participants in a study by Siedlecki et al. (2014). While social support and our ability to form social networks can be very beneficial to one's health and well-being, imbalances may occur, especially when the balance is disturbed by such a strong stressor such as an illness of someone within the social network, and solutions may be hard to come by.

A cancer diagnosis for a member of a social network can be one of the most socially disrupting events that they, their family, and their friend may ever experience. At the same time however, it is when the survivor needs social support the most. They may become reclusive and try to distance themselves from those around them, embarrassed of the toll the illness has taken on their body and depressed about the uncertainty of their condition. Those who may have been once active members of their community, be it whether by volunteering, being employed, being active in their religious community, staying active in sports and recreation, or simply actively being a part of their friends and family's lives may choose to no longer be as proactive in their social engagements. Their loved ones may try their best to try and maintain normalcy in the survivor's social life in vain and become increasingly frustrated and may even recluse themselves from social engagements as well. While the survivor may be seen in the clinical setting weekly or monthly for a few hours, there is a huge amount of time where they are not around health care professionals and it is in this time period where all they have to rely on is their social support.

A study by Wright et al. (2002) sought to evaluate and categorize the social problems experienced by cancer patients throughout treatment. They identified 32 social problems and categorized them under eight headings, managing in the home, health and welfare services, finances, employment, legal matters, relationships and, sexuality and body image (Wright et al. 2002). The results of the study determined a statistically significant proportion of participants experienced problems in every single category.

While the theory behind social support, social networks, social involvement, and so on in the life of a cancer survivor is all sound, what remains is probably the hardest part; trying to put the theory to practice. Helping a cancer survivor return to normalcy in their social lives seems much easier in theory than it does in practice.

Psychosocial Problems in Esophageal Cancer Patients

Psychosocial problems are especially rampant in patients with esophageal cancer due to a variety of factors. In fact, rate of psychological illness in esophageal cancer patients is higher than rates reported for others such as breast, prostate, bronchial, and gastrointestinal cancers (Dempster et al. 2011). Why is psychological illness so common in esophageal cancer patients specifically? In a study by Vodermaier et al. (2009), which encompassed patients with a variety of different cancers, it was found that rates of psychological illness were most elevated in patients suffering from late-stage illnesses, with a poor prognosis, requiring invasive surgery, all elements common to esophageal cancer patients. Furthermore, study by Bergquist et al. (2007) 42 % of esophageal cancer patients studied exhibited symptoms of depression within 2 years of diagnosis and 34 % of patients showed anxiety symptoms within the same time frame. Both numbers are indeed higher than depression or anxiety statistics for patients with other forms of gastrointestinal cancers. Esophageal cancer patients were also shown the be the most at-risk population for suicide and death from cardiovascular causes upon diagnosis, in a study of over six million newly diagnosed cancer patients, indicating the magnitude of the stressor at diagnosis with the disease can be (Fang et al. 2012).

To the psychological tribulations placed upon the patient, esophageal cancer can strain a patient's social relationships as well. The dysphagia, or problems swallowing, which the majority of patients experience before and after treatment, cause many problems at the interpersonal and social level. In patients who have undergone esophagectomy, the stomach is often pushed upwards in the abdomen, shrinking it in size and exacerbating eating discomforts (Wainwright et al. 2007). Patient's feel as if they have little control over how the body will react to eating, as many will simply not be able to swallow their food properly or vomit even if they do. They feel they no longer fit the social norms and expectations governing what might be thought of as acceptable eating behavior. For these reasons, they will often withdraw themselves from eating in the company of friends and family. They isolate themselves for fear of embarrassing themselves at the table, showing their social circle how affected they are by their disease (Wainwright et al. 2007).

Family and close friends will also be forced to assume an active role in helping, and caring for their loved one. This places a good amount of responsibility and stress on the caregiver, who themselves feel overwhelmed with the amount of support the patients need. In turn, psychological distress strikes the caregiver as well, leading to feelings of depression and anxiety (Wainwright et al. 2007).

Psychosocial Interventions: Social Workers and Oncologists

Oncology social work as a profession is relatively new having been established in the 1970s (Fobair 2009). The Association of Oncology Social Workers defines the profession as "designed to promote the patient's best utilization of the health care system, the optimal development of coping strategies and the mobilization of community resources to support maximum functioning" (Fobair 2009). For the time the survivor spends outside of the clinic, social workers are, for the most part, one of the only resources the survivor and their family has for helping to cope with their day-to-day services and helping to steer end-of-life-care when needed. Social workers provide the survivor with practical assistance for home care, transportation and access to counseling and support groups. They will also provide respite services to family members and friends who themselves will go through trying times attempting to support and be available for their ill loved one.

Nevertheless, the power of social support groups, (which may include cancer survivors) and inter-family comfort cannot be understated. For example, a buddy-system via the telephone that would be available 24 h a day to answer concerns and questions providing caregivers with added reassurance. Patients, and their families, have a firsthand experience of what it means to cope with esophageal cancer, and helping educate other families on the matter is extremely helpful. Patients and families taking solace in the fact that they are not alone in the fight helps as well. Physicians at the Mayo Clinic in Florida recently debuted a social network connecting esophageal cancer patients and their families from across the globe. The head of this initiative, Herbert Wolfsen, M.D., explains that connecting esophageal cancer patients and their families fills the gap in knowledge which most health care professionals have about actually having to live with the disease. "Physicians can talk about the technical aspects of esophageal cancer and its treatment, but we don't really know what it means to have issues with breathing, eating, sleeping, and just trying to live a normal life after cancer treatment, because we haven't had this experience. We understand more about the many issues that our patients can really struggle to overcome. Many of the techniques, methods, medications, and lifestyles changes they develop to cope with them aren't in the textbooks—they are word of mouth," he says (Mayo Clinic Esophageal Cancer Patients Support Each Other Through Facebook Group 2011) "Nothing works the same for each person, and every patient's experience is valuable" (Mayo Clinic 2011). These forms of support groups can be invaluable and should be encouraged to all patient families.

Nutritional Interventions

While all cancer patients constitute as an at-risk population for nutrition related complications, esophageal cancer survivors face unique challenges in trying to maintain adequate nutrition (Miller and Bozeman 2012). The nature of the illness brings with it very specific barriers to adequate feeding which nutritionists, doctors and nurses must consider when guiding the patient through treatment. While maintaining adequate nutrition may not seem to be of primary importance in a cancer survivor's treatment, its value towards the survivor's prognosis and HRQoL cannot be understated. "[Adequate nutrition] helps in controlling cancer-related symptoms, reduces postoperative complications and infection rate, shortens length of the hospital stay, improves tolerance to treatment, and enhances immunometabolic host response." (Marin Caro et al. 2007). Further research specific to esophageal cancer survivors who have undergone esophagectomy has concluded that perioperative nutrition status can be taken as an independent indicator for prognosis after surgery and chances for complications (Filip et al. 2015). The study concluded patients with insufficient nutrition scores were more likely to suffer from severe complications.

The volatility of a cancer survivor's nutrition status is a well-characterized risk factor. While the nutrition needs of a healthy, average body mass individual are as simple as matching energy intake with energy expenditure, the nutrition needs of a cancer survivor are markedly more complex. The effects of a malignant growth anywhere in the body are felt on numerous biochemical and physiological body pathways, a syndrome known as cancer cachexia (Tisdale 2009). The nature of esophageal malignancies makes feeding all the more challenging, as swallowing is a challenge for the vast majority of patients, before and after treatment.

Cancer cachexia is the syndrome which common to survivors of all classes of cancers. More than 50 % of all cancer survivors suffer from symptoms of this syndrome, notably progressive weight loss, loss of appetite, early satiety and atrophy of the body's skeletal muscle mass (Tisdale 2009). Esophageal cancer patients suffer from cachexia at one of the highest incidence rates, along with gastric cancer, and pancreatic cancer survivors (Tisdale 2009).

Nutritional issues for cancer patients are complex enough, but the nature of esophageal cancer unfortunately exacerbates these problems and causes them to be more difficult to treat. As already discussed, the vast majority of esophageal cancer patients present to the clinic with existing dysphagia and trouble feeding due to the malignancy occluding the esophageal lumen. Many patients enter the clinic having lost weight in recent months. Treatments are a double-edged sword, as feeding becomes more difficult and additional stressors are placed on the body inducing stress responses and additional energy requirements. Surgery, depending on the type of procedure and anatomy of the tumor, may worsen the dysphagia for a period after surgery due to the scaring and healing at the site of resection (Schoeff et al. 2013). The perioperative period is also hard on the patient, with the anxiety and pain adding to the difficulties. Chemotherapy inherently affects the lining of the gastrointestinal tract leading to possible mucositis, enteritis and ulcerations, as well as the immune system, leading to increased rate of infections and increased metabolic rate (Miller and Bozeman 2012). Radiotherapy of the esophagus also brings with it a gamut of side effects making the passage of food difficult (Miller and Bozeman 2012). While these treatments may in the end be successful in alleviating dysphagia, the patients will first have to pass through a harsh period. It is of no surprise that 60–85 % of esophageal cancer survivors are reported to be malnourished at some time during treatment (Gupta and Ihmaidat 2003). One study reported 90 % of esophageal cancer patients were malnourished at their first visit to the clinic (Silvers et al. 2014). While all cancer patients constitute as an at-risk population for malnutrition, esophageal cancer patients are even more vulnerable.

Malnourishment in esophageal cancer patients has a serious impact on a patient's prognosis and quality of life. Malnourishment during esophageal cancer treatment has been shown to decrease the effectiveness of chemotherapy and radiation treatments, aggravate the side effects of said treatments and negatively impact prognosis and quality of life (Bollschweiler et al. 2013).

Nutritional Interventions in Esophageal Cancer Patients

The care of a dietician with a plan tailored for each and every patient is invaluable to the prognosis and HRQoL for every esophageal cancer survivor. Two studies investigated the effects of having patients undergo intensive nutritional intervention before and throughout treatment. Ligthart-Melis et al. (2012) reported esophageal cancer patients receiving nutritional support via a dietician regularly before and after surgery had significantly reduced rates of postoperative complications and length of stay in the ICU compared with patients who had not received such counseling 3 years prior to the study. Silvers et al. (2014) had a dietician counsel patients at the time of diagnosis. Patients receiving tailored consultations had decreased weight loss, decreased nutritional risk scores, and increased HRQoL scores compared with baseline before and after treatment. The ideal nutrition treatment starts at the time of diagnosis, by assessing the patient's nutritional status.

Doctors, nurses, and dieticians collaborate depending on the patient's dysphagia score, based on a Likert scale of 0–4 (Sharma and Kozarek 2009). Further considerations are taken,

0	Able to consume a normal diet
1	Dysphagia with certain solid foods
2	Able to swallow semi-solid soft foods
3	Able to swallow liquids only
4	Unable to swallow saliva (complete dysphagia)

such as any recent weight loss, nausea, vomiting, diarrhea, or constipation.

Commentary from a nutritionist:

> I see them in the clinic where there is an "eating dysfunction," weight loss, progression from inability to eat solids, to softer foods, to liquids. The time frame for this progression is variable from weeks to months but it is not uncommon to see them only be able to get down an 8 oz. bottle of Ensure, once a day.

Until treatment can be started, the dietician can only intervene to a certain extent. They will council the patient on trying to choose the right foods, which have the right texture, but are also the most nutrient and calorie dense. The best feeding plan is to eat very small meals every 1–2 h. Some patients in this pre-treatment, post-diagnosis phase often try to override the signals the body is giving them and try to force themselves back into a state of "normality" by consuming their typical food in normal portions, which leads to regurgitation, and/or nausea and/or vomiting. Others will react completely in the opposite way, and will develop strong dislike for food and the ill-feelings it brings that they will cease feeding altogether (Wainwright et al. 2007). All patients are still adjusting to food no longer being pleasurable and becoming more of a fixation and a chore. Every feeding period brings with it a reminder that they are no longer healthy, creating an aversion to feeding. While treatment has not even started, nutrition for these patients is essential for withstanding future treatments and helping with prognosis.

After diagnosis, the patient may be admitted to hospital for surgery if the dysphagia is very severe, or they will be sent for chemotherapy and/or radiotherapy. Patients immediately admitted may require alternative feeding methods to oral feeding, either via an enteral feeding tube, a gastrostomy or a jejunostomy (Allum et al. 2011). However, if treatment can be initiated rapidly, chemotherapy with effective agents is generally associated with a rapid improvement in their swallowing and may gain weight in this time period (Cools-Lartigue et al., Annals of Surgical Oncology 2015). Granted there are many side effects of chemotherapy, but compared with their baseline, their HRQoL improves in these 6–8 weeks post-diagnosis, after neo-adjuvant therapy (preoperative), surgery, and adjuvant therapy (postoperative). The tumor has now shrunk significantly due to the chemotherapy and they begin their path to recover. Patients who must receive both chemotherapy and radiotherapy generally experience a great deal of pain and often require the help of alternative feeding methods to get through this active and aggressive treatment phase.

Nursing and Physician Interventions

Oncology nurses practice in a variety of settings, including home health care agencies, acute care hospitals, ambulatory care clinics, private oncologist's offices and radiation therapy and chemotherapy facilities. While the settings may be numerous and varied, the role of nurses in the care of esophageal cancer patients is very often involving direct patient care. From patient assessment, to patient education, symptom management and coordination and planning of treatment, nurses are one of the key cogs in a patient's battle with cancer.

The initial role for oncology nurses dealing with esophageal cancer patients is a triage of their situation. They first assess a patient's Eastern Cooperative Oncology Group (ECOG) Performance Status, a measurement of the degree to which the disease has affected the patient's ability to perform their daily activities. The nurse will then assess the patient's resources in terms of support groups. The support group survivors often include family and friends, who will be able to provide additional moral and physical support, which is needed throughout the treatment trajectory. Two studies by Allison and Edgar (2005–2009) highlighted the effectiveness of a coping strategy intervention for people with head and next cancer (including esophageal cancer patients). Allison et al. (2004) also found that a psycho-educational intervention was useful in providing psychosocial support to individuals with head and neck cancer.

Conclusions and Future Perspectives

Sir William Osler often considered to be the "father of modern medicine" for his work done demonstrating the importance of bedside manner in the clinic, once said "The good physician treats the disease, the great physician treats the patient with the disease" (Centor 2007, p. 59). The essence of this statement embodies the aim of this chapter in many regards. This chapter provided an overview of the current state of esophageal cancer management through the lenses of various health care professionals, whether physicians, nurses, social workers, or psychosocial oncologists, yet all the while focused upon how their work improves a patient's quality of life through their battle with an incredibly devastating disease which oftentimes surpasses most other cancers in regard to detriment upon various aspects of a patient's HRQoL. In simpler terms, the chapter addressed the human aspect of cancer survivorship, beyond basic science and clinical treatment.

One could read journals and books about cancer for many years and still not be close to wading through the existing literature on the disease, which only continues to grow. Simply typing "cancer" into the PubMed Database search bar provides 3.1 million articles on the subject. Similar increases in article numbers are seen in articles dealing with esophageal cancer. The literature pool on every type is expanding at an incredible rate, with new discoveries in the field made every day. However, we must try and maintain a balance between viewing and treating a patient. This is why quality of life scores are so important, and why the therapeutic interventions mentioned in this chapter to maximize their quality of life are so crucial.

Esophageal cancer treatment in the clinic, in the home, in cancer support centers, and elsewhere, is performed by professionals who have decades of research, training, and experience. In the clinic, everything from chemotherapy doses and choice of drugs to surgical techniques and precision to perioperative care, the work of physicians and nurses with esophageal cancer patients cannot be understated. The social workers that enter the homes and communities of these patients and provide individualized support to each based on their social situation, finances, and morale are able to help patients by removing some of the burden of cancer from the patient and their families. And finally the psychosocial oncologists who are able to work with cancer survivors by supporting their mental health through a disease, could cause burn-out among even the toughest of characters.

While 5-year survival rates in the 1960s and 1970s dwindled in the 5 % range, rates have improved to estimates from 20 % (Gaur et al. 2014) to 39 % (American Association for Thoracic Surgery 2015). Similar to all cancers however, the best chance of survival is to detect the malignancy at an early stage from routine colonoscopies and mammograms. Routine endoscopies, or the insertion of a viewing camera into the esophagus, have been proposed, especially for the most at-risk population such as patients with GERD and/or mild dysphagia but the cost-effectiveness of this plan is unrealistic to health care centers (Gaur et al. 2014).

Furthermore, we hope that this chapter will provide increased awareness about esophageal cancer, as recent epidemiological data is alarming. These trends are alarming and coupled with the low 5-year survival rates and the high impact on a patient's quality of life, the disease should garner even greater attention among all health care professionals.

Acknowledgments This author wishes to acknowledge the ongoing support and assistance from Mary Diovisalvi, RN—Pivot Nurse in Upper GI Cancer—McGill University Hospital Center (MUHC), and Eleanor Eckert—Nutritionist in Upper GI Cancer—MUHC.

References

Abrams, J. A. (2009). Are we making progress in preventing Barrett's-related esophageal cancer? *Therapeutic Advances in Gastroenterology*, *2*(2), 73–77. doi:10.1177/1756283X08102044

Ajani, J. A., Barthel, J. S., Bentrem, D. J., D'Amico, T. A., Das, P., Denlinger, C. S., et al. (2011). Esophageal and esophagogastric junction cancers. *Journal of the National Comprehensive Cancer Network: JNCCN*, *8*, 830–887.

Alexandre, L., Long, E., & Beales, I. L. (2014). Pathophysiological mechanisms linking obesity and esophageal adenocarcinoma. *World Journal of Gastrointestinal Pathophysiology, 5*(4), 534–549. doi:10.4291/wjgp.v5.i4.534

Allison, P.J., (PI) & Edgar, L. (Co-PI) (2005–2009). A randomized control trial of the Effectiveness of a coping strategy intervention for people with head and next cancer (Canadian Institute for Health Research (CIHR).

Allison, P. J., Edgar, L., Black, M., & Heir, M. (2004). Results of a feasibility study for a psycho-educational intervention in head and neck cancer. *Journal of Psycho-Oncology, 13,* 482–485.

Allum, W. H., Blazeby, J. M., Griffin, S. M., Cunningham, D., Jankowski, J. A., & Wong, R. (2011). Guidelines for the management of oesophageal and gastric cancer. *Gut, 11*, 1449–1472.

Bergquist, H., Ruth, M., & Hammerlid, E. (2007). Psychiatric morbidity among patients with cancer of the esophagus or the gastro-esophageal junction: A prospective, longitudinal evaluation. *Diseases of the Esophagus: Official Journal of the International Society for Diseases of the Esophagus/I.S.D.E, 6,* 523–529.

Bollschweiler, E., Herbold, T., Plum, P., & Holscher, A. H. (2013). Prognostic relevance of nutritional status in patients with advanced esophageal cancer. *Expert Review of Anticancer Therapy, 3*, 275–278.

Canadian Cancer Society's Advisory Committee on Cancer Statistics. (2015, June 6). *Canadian cancer statistics 2015*. Toronto, ON: Canadian Cancer Society. Cancer Research UK. "Men are 50 per cent more likely to get esophageal cancer than 30 years ago." *Science Daily*.

Centor, R. M. (2007). To be a great physician, you must understand the whole story. *Medscape General Medicine, 9*(1), 59.

Cools-Lartigue, J., Spicer, J., & Ferri, L. E. (2015). Current status of management of malignant disease: current management of esophageal cancer. *Journal of Gastrointestinal Surgery: Official Journal of the Society for Surgery of the Alimentary Tract, 5*, 964–972.

Darling, G. E. (2013). Quality of life in patients with esophageal cancer. *Thoracic Surgery Clinics, 4*, 569–575.

Dempster, M., McCorry, N. K., Brennan, E., Donnelly, M., Murray, L., & Johnston, B. T. (2011). Psychological distress among survivors of esophageal cancer: the role of illness cognitions and coping. *Diseases of the Esophagus: Official Journal of the International Society for Diseases of the Esophagus/I.S.D.E, 3,* 222–227.

DeVita, V., Lawrence, T., & Rosenberg, S. (Eds.). (2008). *DeVita, Hellman, & Rosenberg's cancer: Principles & practice of oncology* (8th ed.). Philadelphia: Wolters Kluwer/Lippincott Williams & Wilkins.

Djarv, T., Lagergren, J., Blazeby, J. M., & Lagergren, P. (2008). Long-term health-related quality of life following surgery for oesophageal cancer. *The British Journal of Surgery, 9*, 1121–1126.

Fang, F., Fall, K., Mittleman, M. A., Sparen, P., Ye, W., Adami, H. O., et al. (2012). Suicide and cardiovascular death after a cancer diagnosis. *The New England Journal of Medicine, 14*, 1310–1318.

Filip, B., Scarpa, M., Cavallin, F., Cagol, M., Alfieri, R., Saadeh, L., et al. (2015). Postoperative outcome after oesophagectomy for cancer: Nutritional status is the missing ring in the current prognostic scores. *European Journal of Surgical Oncology: The Journal of the European Society of Surgical Oncology and the British Association of Surgical Oncology, 6*, 787–794.

Fobair, P. (2009). Historical threads in the development of oncology social work. *Journal of Psychosocial Oncology, 27*(2), 155–215. doi:10.1080/07347330902775301

Gaur, P., Kim, M. P., & Dunkin, B. J. (2014). Esophageal cancer: Recent advances in screening, targeted therapy, and management. *Journal of Carcinogenesis,* 11.

Gottlieb, B. H., & Bergen, A. E. (2009). Social support concepts and measures. *Journal of Psychosomatic Research, 5*, 511–520.

Gupta, R., & Ihmaidat, H. (2003). Nutritional effects of oesophageal, gastric and pancreatic carcinoma. *European Journal of Surgical Oncology, 29*(8), 634–643.

Kypriotakis, G., Vidrine, D. J., Francis, L. E., & Rose, J. H. (2015, May 8). The longitudinal relationship between quality of life and survival in advanced stage cancer. *Psycho-Oncology*. doi:10.1002/pon.3846 [Epub ahead of print].

Ligthart-Melis, G. C., Weijs, P. J., te Boveldt, N. D., Buskermolen, S., Earthman, C. P., Verheul, H. M., de Lange-de Klerk, E. S., van Weyenberg, S. J., & van der Peet, D. L. (2012). Dietician-delivered intensive nutritional support is associated with a decrease in severe postoperative complications after surgery in patients with esophageal cancer. *Diseases of the Esophagus: Official Journal of the International Society for Diseases of the Esophagus/ I.S.D.E, 6*, 587–593.

Marin Caro, M. M., Laviano, A., & Pichard, C. (2007). Nutritional intervention and quality of life in adult oncology patients. *Clinical nutrition (Edinburgh, Scotland), 3,* 289–301.

Mayo Clinic Esophageal Cancer Patients Support Each Other Through Facebook Group (2011). Press Release Distribution, EDGAR Filing, XBRL, Regulatory Filings. Business Wire. Retrieved April 22 2016.

McNair, A. G., Brookes, S. T., Kinnersley, P., & Blazeby, J. M. (2013). What surgeons should tell patients with oesophago-gastric cancer: A cross sectional study of information needs. *European Journal of Surgical Oncology: The Journal of the European Society of Surgical Oncology and the British Association of Surgical Oncology, 11*, 1278–1286.

Mescher, A., & Junqueira, L. (2013). Digestive tract. In *Junqueira's basic histology: Text and atlas* (13th ed.). New York: McGraw-Hill.

Miller, K. R., & Bozeman, M. C. (2012). Nutrition therapy issues in esophageal cancer. *Current gastroenterology reports, 14*, 356–366.

Patel, K., Wakhisi, J., Mining, S., Mwangi, A., & Patel, R. (2013). Esophageal cancer, the topmost cancer at MTRH in the Rift Valley, Kenya, and its potential risk factors. *ISRN oncology, 2013*, Article ID 503249, 9 p. doi:10.1155/2013/5032495

Rab, F (2012). Social support as a determinant of health related quality of life in breast cancer survivors in California. Electronic Thesis and Dissertation Repository. Paper 871.S.

Rustgi, A. K., & El-Serag, H. B. (2014). Esophageal carcinoma. *The New England Journal of Medicine, 26*, 2499–2509.

Schlansky, B., Dimarino, A. J., Loren, D., Infantolino, A., Kowalski, T., & Cohen, S. (2006). A survey of oesophageal cancer: Pathology, stage and clinical presentation. *Alimentary Pharmacology & Therapeutics, 5*, 587–593

Schoeff, S. S., Barrett, D. M., Gress, C. D., & Jameson, M. J. (2013). Nutritional management for head and neck cancer patients. *Nutrition Issues in Practical Gastroenterology, 121*, 43–51.

Schulz, R., & Beach, S. R. (1999). Caregiving as a risk factor for mortality: The caregiver health effects study. *Journal of American Medical Association, 23*, 2215–2219.

SEER Stat Fact Sheets: Esophageal Cancer. (2015). Retrieved from http://seer.cancer.gov/statfacts/html/esoph.html

Sharma, P., & Kozarek, R. (2009). Role of esophageal stents in benign and malignant diseases. *The American Journal of Gastroenterology, 2,* 258–273. quiz 274.

Siedlecki, K. L., Salthouse, T. A., Oishi, S., & Jeswani, S. (2014). The relationship between social support and subjective well-being across age. *Social Indicators Research, 2*, 561–576.

Silvers, M. A., Savva, J., Huggins, C. E., Truby, H., & Haines, T. (2014). Potential benefits of early nutritional intervention in adults with upper gastrointestinal cancer: A pilot randomised trial. *Supportive Care in Cancer: Official Journal of the Multinational Association of Supportive Care in Cancer, 11*, 3035–3044.

Talley, N., DeVault, K., & Fleischer, D. (Eds.). (2010). *Practical gastroenterology and hepatology esophagus and stomach*. Somerset: Wiley.

Tisdale, M. J. (2009). Mechanisms of cancer cachexia. *Physiological Reviews, 2*, 381–410.

Torre, L. A., Bray, F., Siegel, R. L., Ferlay, J., Lortet-Tieulent, J., & Jemal, A. (2015). Global cancer statistics, 2012. *CA: A Cancer Journal for Clinicians, 2*, 87–8108.

Trask, P. C., Hsu, M. A., & McQuellon, R. (2009). Other paradigms: health-related quality of life as a measure in cancer treatment: Its importance and relevance. *Cancer Journal (Sudbury, Mass.), 5*, 435–440.

Vodermaier, A., Linden, W., & Siu, C. (2009). Screening for emotional distress in cancer patients: A systematic review of assessment instruments. *Journal of the National Cancer Institute, 21*, 1464–1488.

Wainwright, D., Donovan, J. L., Kavadas, V., Cramer, H., & Blazeby, J. M. (2007). Remapping the body: Learning to eat again after surgery for esophageal cancer. *Qualitative Health Research, 6*, 759–771.

What are the key statistics about cancer of the esophagus? (2014, March 20). Retrieved July 13, 2015. Retrieved from http://www.cancer.org/cancer/esophaguscancer/detailedguide/esophagus-cancer-key-statistics

Wright, E. P., Kiely, M. A., Lynch, P., Cull, A., & Selby, P. J. (2002). Social problems in oncology. *British Journal of Cancer, 10*, 1099–1104.

Chapter 10
The Family Caregiver as Cancer Survivor: Supporting and Promoting Positive Bereavement Outcomes

Lorraine Holtslander

Introduction

Bereaved family caregivers are rarely seen as cancer survivors, however, the experience of being a caregiver for a family member with advanced cancer will no doubt leave them as a cancer survivor of an often intense and overwhelming illness experience. The Canadian Hospice Palliative Care Association (CHPCA) recognizes that family caregivers also experience the illness and death of the person they are caring for and must embark on a significant transition as they enter into bereavement (CHPCA 2013). Family caregivers while being extensively relied upon by the health care system during the cancer journey are often left to face bereavement without support, often after enduring an exhausting and difficult caregiving experience. Their experiences as caregivers can greatly affect their bereavement journey and not all will experience positive outcomes. Very little is known about how to assess those at most risk of negative outcomes nor which supports should be offered. This chapter will examine new evidence for caregiver support initiatives that facilitate the need for a comprehensive assessment and an individualized approach that considers how diverse their experience often is. This is an underresourced global concern as the world is facing a growing number of cancer deaths due to an increasing and aging population (World Health Organization 2015). There is an urgent need to develop interventions that support family caregivers during the process of caregiving for an advanced cancer patient, including their bereavement. Family caregivers must be recognized as part of the

L. Holtslander (✉)
College of Nursing, University of Saskatchewan,
4216 E Wing Health Science Bldg, 104 Clinic Place, Saskatoon
SK S7N 2Z4, Canada
e-mail: lorraine.holtslander@usask.ca

L. Holtslander
University of the Witwatersrand, Johannesburg, South Africa

T.R. Fitzpatrick (ed.), *Treating Vulnerable Populations of Cancer Survivors: A Biopsychosocial Approach*, DOI 10.1007/978-3-319-32364-0_10

spectrum of cancer survivorship in order to support global health and avoid a public health crisis.

Background

The processes of bereavement itself has a negative effect on overall morbidity and mortality of caregivers (Stroebe et al. 2007), including a risk of suicide (Erlangsen et al. 2004), complicated grief and depression (Holtslander and McMillan 2011), loneliness, substance abuse, physical and emotional illnesses (Schulz et al. 2008), pain and physical distress (Kowalski and Bondmass 2008), sleep disturbance (Carter 2005), and even death (Christakis and Iwashyna 2003). The need to support bereaved caregivers is urgent and growing, as deaths from cancer will continue to rise dramatically across the world. The Canadian Cancer Society predicts that cancer deaths will increase by 79 % by 2028 and the number of new cancer cases will more than double in those ages 65 and over (Canadian Cancer Statistics 2015). This is due primarily to an aging population, population growth and an increased risk of cancer, but these demographic changes will have a huge impact on the demand and the need for services and supports around the world. Even though family caregivers are relied upon to sustain already overwhelmed health care systems, many more family caregivers will be required, affecting the lives of many individuals, families and communities. However, very little is known about how best to identify those at most risk of complicated grief, and which supports and services are most effective.

The term "secondary survivor" has been used to describe a family member or caregiver who has been impacted by the cancer experience (Clark et al. 2011). Secondary survivors described feeling vulnerable, emanating from a loss of control and a sense of alienation from the team providing care to the patient, which affected them into bereavement. However, it is worthwhile to recognize that bereaved family caregivers have indeed "survived" the cancer experience, considering the caregiving that was required, as well as the ultimate loss of a family member to cancer. In many situations, their lives are completely changed, resulting in overwhelming physical, emotional and social needs as they both recover from the exhaustion of caregiving and often face a new life without a partner (Holtslander et al. 2011). In most cases, these are older adults, in particular women who have lost a spouse, presenting with a particular risk of health concerns, loneliness and immense challenges in reconstructing their identity after caregiving (Naef et al. 2013). Specifically the cancer experience has been associated with worse outcomes, such as being a caregiver to a person with lung or ovarian cancer. Often there is such difficult symptom management that caregivers reported being traumatized and in shock by the experience of caring for a person with ovarian cancer (Sanderson et al. 2013). Caregivers of persons with lung cancer reported ill health and suffering in physical, social, psychological, and spiritual realms as a result of their caregiving experiences (Ellis 2012).

Despite current national and international standards for palliative care that include the provision of a support system to help the family cope during the patient's illness and continuing into their own bereavement (World Health Organization 2002), very little is known about how best to support family caregivers as they transition into bereavement. The Canadian Hospice Palliative Care Association (2013) recognizes that family members are affected by the illness of the patient and that the bereavement process must be supported in order to achieve a positive, healing transition, rebuild their lives and reintegrate into society. Both caregiving and bereavement are becoming imperative public health issues, as caregivers themselves may become patients and struggle to fulfill their multiple responsibilities at home and in the workplace (2013). Specifically, bereaved family caregivers often struggled to find balance in their emotions and thoughts after caregiving ends, as they make sense of their caregiving experiences and face life that requires a new purpose (Holtslander and Duggleby 2009).

Metasynthesis and Qualitative Research

In order to identify the most appropriate supports, policies and interventions specific to bereaved caregivers, a rigorous metasynthesis of qualitative research with bereaved caregivers of an advanced cancer patient, who had received palliative care, was completed by the author and her team. Although the search procedures and overall results are reported elsewhere (Holtslander et al. in process) this chapter will highlight practical applications of the key themes identified, including the challenging emotions and mental health concerns, a lack of support, and the need for follow-up including an assessment of those most at risk and how to offer specific interventions.

In total there were 22 qualitative studies included in the metasynthesis, representing eight countries (Canada, Australia, USA, N. Ireland, Hong Kong, Japan, Sweden and England). The total number of bereaved caregiver participants was 375, including 222 women and 108 men, when reported. All of these studies described and interpreted the loss, grief, and bereavement experience of caregivers of a cancer patient, which was contextually very complex and diverse for each individual. Specific assessment and interventions can be developed based on these findings, as factors were identified that helped each individual to move forward through their loss while identifying those factors that may cause difficulty and predispose to prolonged or complicated grief.

"Honoring the voices" of bereaved caregivers was the goal of the metasynthesis of qualitative research. Qualitative research provides the best source of evidence for research and practice since it has been conducted in the real world and not a laboratory (Sandelowski and Barroso 2007). Key themes from a metasynthesis of qualitative research with bereaved caregivers of an advanced cancer patient who received palliative care that offer the most practical guidance for assessment and intervention will be presented. Key areas of assessment and specific focus on practical interventions will be included.

Themes from the Metasynthesis of Qualitative Research with Bereaved Caregivers Overwhelming Grief Accompanied by Stressful Thoughts and Emotions

Bereaved caregivers consistently described their experiences after the death of the patient as dealing with many overwhelming and unpredictable emotions (Holtslander and Duggleby 2010), including feelings of disbelief, numbness and regret (Grbich et al. 2001; Hudson 2006), leaving them to cope by living day to day as a result of all-consuming waves of grief (Steeves 2002). Other strong emotions included yearning for the deceased (Asai et al. 2010) and feelings of loneliness and emptiness (Dean et al. 2005; Holtslander et al. 2011). Besides losing someone close to them, caregivers of an advanced cancer patient often are faced with extreme symptom management, and described the "severe shock" and trauma of caregiving (Koop and Strang 2003; Sanderson et al. 2013) as they remembered dealing with the pain and suffering, extreme physical decline, and distressing, intrusive memories of the last few days and weeks of the patient's life. In many situations an extremely close relationship is formed during caregiving, resulting in an even stronger and intense missing of the person who had died and a longing for them to be alive (Stajduhar et al. 2010). Bereaved caregivers often described their feelings of guilt and regrets about caregiving, wishing they had done more as caregivers (Holtslander et al. 2011; Hudson 2006). Family caregivers reported feeling devastated at having let their family member down, specifically facing the impact of "shattered promises" when they were unable to care for the patient at home as promised (Topf et al. 2013). This range of very difficult emotions often led to specific mental health concerns and bereaved caregivers felt a loss of confidence in their ability to look forward beyond a day-to-day existence (Grbich et al. 2001).

Specific Mental Health Issues Arising from Bereavement

A surprising number of mental health issues predominated when caregivers were asked about their experiences, even though this was not a focus of the studies, and was often an exclusion criteria for participating. Bereaved caregivers expressed their anger at the person who had died (Stajduhar et al. 2010), anger for being left (Sanderson et al. 2013), and anger about the death itself (Chan and Chan 2011; Hegge 1991). Bereaved caregivers commonly reported anxiety, confusion and worry about the future (Asai et al. 2010), difficulty coping and panic attacks (Hudson 2006). Some had difficulty accepting that their loved one has passed away. This included carrying on as though they were still there, "this is not happening" feelings, and not accepting the reality of the loss (Asai et al. 2010). Sometimes this included not attending memorial services or delayed grieving. Of real concern is that some of the bereaved caregivers' reported feelings of hopelessness (Holtslander and Duggleby 2010), even to the point of considering suicide (Agnew et al. 2008) which was reported in a study where the diagnosis of a mental illness was an exclusion criterion, as well depression and panic attacks were commonly described. Bereaved caregivers struggled with finding purpose or meaning (Holtslander and Duggleby 2009; Sanderson et al. 2013), a lack of direction (Grbich et al. 2001), and feeling unable to cope, dazed and confused (Hudson 2006). These mental health issues are of great concern since bereaved caregivers will face many negative physical, social and emotional consequences if not addressed.

Lack of Support: Social Isolation and Loneliness

Most of the samples of participants in the metasynthesis of research with bereaved caregivers were older women who had cared for a spouse; commonly resulting in overwhelming loneliness and the loss of a companion to share day-to-day life (Agnew et al. 2008; Chan and Chan 2011; Holtslander and Duggleby 2010). Caregiving itself may have been an isolating experience, as caregivers become consumed with their duties and unable to maintain connection with their usual support networks (Stajduhar et al. 2010). A common experience during bereavement was social isolation and loneliness (Asai et al. 2010), and a great deal of worry about a future alone, with no one to look after them (Holtslander and Duggleby 2010). Being unexpectedly single after having established a strong lifetime partnership resulted in a great deal of uncertainty in the future (Hornjatkevyc 2011) and the absence of a trusted confidant (Hegge 1991). In a study of caregivers who had cared for an adult child with cancer, social isolation was also a finding, as their family and friends and coworkers people were often uncomfortable with the sort of grief they were uniquely experiencing (Dean et al. 2005). Family and friends were essential and reported as the main sources of support in most of the studies, but often these individuals were also grieving in their own way and each experienced the loss differently (Agnew et al. 2008). The support of religious networks (Grbich et al. 2001) and finding professional and counseling support was also identified as essential (Dean et al. 2005; Hornjatkevyc 2011). Although many hospice programs reported offering bereavement support, many declined such support, describing the stigma of accepting professional support or a reluctance to share in a group (Agnew et al. 2008; Dean et al. 2005). Bereaved caregivers may also be reluctant to ask for help (Dumont et al. 2008) or feeling a sense of distance from others (Pusa et al. 2012), so even though social support is essential to surviving such an experience, finding and maintaining these networks is a great challenge.

Assessment: Who Is at the Most Risk for Complicated Grief?

Vignette: Agnes was 87 years old and was happy and proud to be the primary caregiver for her spouse until he died of cancer at the age of 88. At six months after his death, Agnes was having a difficult time, as she reflected on life alone after 60 years of marriage: "I feel like someone chopped one of my arms off." While focusing her time and attention on caring for her husband, Agnes had neglected her own symptoms of a worsening heart condition. The couple's one child lived out of town and their family support system was very limited both during caregiving and into bereavement. Their daughter was also exhausted from traveling to support her parents and needed to attend to her own family during the bereavement phase of the palliative care journey. Agnes finally kept an appointment with her cardiologist. She was admitted to hospital but would never return home. At 7 months after the death of her husband, Agnes died in hospital, unable to recover from the combination of a pre-existing heart condition, the stress and exhaustion of caregiving, and the great many losses she was facing.

In a time of limited health care resources, it is essential to identify those at most risk of complications and offer them the most effective and meaningful support. Qualitative research findings provide strong support for the individual and diverse experience of each situation, yet common factors can be identified that include the need to assess their unique strengths and challenges, combined with the type of loss, the coping strategies being employed, the experience of caregiving itself, and the support systems they have in place. It is essential to identify the specific concerns of each individual, based on both current physical and emotional symptoms and a history of mental health concerns, previous or concurrent losses, and the caregiving roles they were involved in. Qualitative research has shown that the appraisal of the caregiving experience, either as positive or a negative experience, had a huge impact on bereavement outcomes, as many bereaved caregivers continued to question the decisions they made on behalf of the dying patient long after the death (Dean et al. 2005; Dumont et al. 2008; Stajduhar et al. 2010; Topf et al. 2013). An assessment of the caregiving experience including their personal history of physical and emotional health and the support networks that are currently in place is essential. The story of their caregiving experience can reveal many areas of unresolved guilt or regrets. Assessment of the personal value of the caregiving experience will yield valuable insight into how they are making meaning of their caregiving story and how it is impacting their grief and bereavement processes. A discussion of the actual physical caregiving they provided and how it affected them is essential. Assessing the losses they face, such as of their own caregiver, automobile driver, or place to live is all too common with older adults. Also essential is a thorough assessment of support and identifying specific people and agencies they can turn to for meeting their needs. Referrals to professional services and supports may be required.

Intervention: Valuing the Caregiving Experience and Supporting Positive Outcomes

The results of the metasynthesis yielded a startling array of ways to support bereaved caregivers as they find unique ways to move forward in grief and begin to make meaning of a very challenging situation. It is essential to identify the emotions and thoughts being processed by the bereaved caregiver, and if a risk for complicated or prolonged grief is identified, providing referrals to counselors, support groups, or appropriate health care providers, is essential. Bereaved caregivers may have physical health concerns that have not been attended to while caregiving, thus follow-up by their health care provider needs to be encouraged.

For bereaved caregivers, bringing value to the caregiving experience for each individual and how he or she is processing any number of losses and recovering from an exhausting experience is essential. Family caregivers may harbor feelings of anger, guilt or regrets, and may even feel unappreciated and this can cause anger and conflict within a family and with the health care system (Stajduhar et al. 2010). Caregivers may feel they have let their family member down when the experience did not go as planned (Topf et al. 2013). Alternatively, many bereaved caregivers emerge with a great deal of pride and a sense of accomplishment (Asai et al. 2010; Koop and Strang 2003), which needs to be encouraged in the meaning-making process. Listening and supporting conflicting emotions and thoughts, even the traumatic memories, of bereaved caregivers as they reflect on their experiences, are a powerful intervention for caregivers during bereavement. Some may wish to write about their experiences, which has also shown benefit (Holtslander and Duggleby 2008).

The metasynthesis revealed that many caregivers found purpose and meaning in helping others as a way to help them through. Of course, interventions must be based on a careful assessment, considering age, gender, access to services, environment, social support and culture. Appropriate interventions are often those mutually found through a supportive conversation with any health care provider.

Vignette: Sherry provided care for her husband Sam, through his journey with multiple myeloma and together they faced many complex and challenging caregiving obstacles, such as pain, immobility, and eventually total paralysis. Sherry believed they were going to get through this and have many more years together, even though Sam was under palliative care services, she was not prepared for the transition to bereavement that would be required. Sherry described how her losses included losing her partner as well as her life's work as they were in business together, and her very identity, which was well known based on their mutual support of her husband as an artist. Caregiving through Sam's cancer journey brought them even closer together, as Sherry learned how to meet her husband's needs for positioning, transferring, comfort and care and she was consistently his strongest advocate. Facing the reality of her loss was very difficult but Sherry described how she became her own "bereavement intervention," finding new purpose in helping others and surrounding herself with a strong support network.

"I had to reinvent myself" through continuing our work, sharing my experiences with others, and relying on my own inner strength and courage, to rebuild a completely changed life after an exhausting, yet extremely rewarding caregiving experience. As Sherry said: "I had to find a purpose."

Building on the principles of *attachment theory* and how they affect the process of adapting to loss (Bowlby 1980), many theorists and practitioners have consequently embraced the adaptive processes of continuing bonds with the deceased, rather than requiring the relinquishing of them (Silverman and Klass 1996). However, recent research shows that efforts to "*make meaning*" of the loss, through personal, practical, or spiritual terms may be a key element in predicting the role and value of attachment and continuing bonds and whether they are helpful in promoting positive outcomes (Neimeyer 2001). A loss as significant as a close family member to whom you have provided care over a period of time can be very painful and challenging as attachment to the care recipient can grow profoundly. When bereaved persons were able to engage in meaning-making activities following their loss, the role of attachment and continuing bonds was predictive of better grief outcomes (Neimeyer et al. 2006). If a survivor is able to make sense of their loss in personal, practical, existential or spiritual terms, continuing bonds with the deceased can be promoted as positive outcomes are usually the result. An individualized, constructivist approach to meaning-making in supporting the caregiver narrative, provides a way to encourage continuing bonds while making sense of the loss (Neimeyer et al. 2006). Theories of attachment theory and meaning-making support the need for exploring the caregiving story and recognizing the individual nature of each person's experience.

Conclusions

Family caregivers are a unique and vulnerable group of cancer survivors, in terms of the effects of cancer on the whole family and how caregivers continue to be impacted by their experience of cancer. Due to the rising number of cancer deaths across the globe, there is an urgent need to value and consider the caregiving experience and the caregiver's role in cancer care. Bereaved caregivers need to be followed to assess their health and well-being, offer interventions and provide support. They need an opportunity to process the cancer experience, reflect on their role as caregivers and be given an opportunity to find meaning and purpose in their current situation.

The results of the metasynthesis of qualitative research with bereaved caregivers must be considered in the light of which countries participated in these qualitative studies, the methodologies applied and degree of interpretation of the researchers, and the sample or participants in each study. Those bereaved caregivers who were unable to talk about or reflect on their experiences may not have been willing to engage in the research. The bereaved caregivers who are struggling the most may have been least likely to participate, thus the findings of these studies only represent the tip of the iceberg when considering just how much difficulty many bereaved caregivers can find themselves in.

For many bereaved caregivers, who have provided care for a spouse or partner with advanced cancer, caregiving was a life-changing experience, often resulting in an overwhelming number of losses and a great deal of loneliness. Qualitative research, when analyzed using metasynthesis techniques, provides insight into an overwhelming experience of grief, specific and concerning mental health issues, the need to recover from the stress of caregiving, and the vital importance of assessment and supportive interventions to promote positive outcomes for this undervalued and often neglected population of cancer survivors. Currently, most bereavement research is not being applied in clinical practice (Hudson 2013), however, a metasynthesis is a powerful tool to base relevant changes to practice by bringing together the results and increasing their combined contribution (Sandelowski and Barroso 2007).

Implications for Clinical Practice

The number of family caregivers will continue to increase with the aging of the population, higher life expectancies, and a shift from institutionalized care to community-based care. Many factors can affect the health and bereavement outcomes of family caregivers such as gender, age, location, education, environment, social support, access to health services, socioeconomic status, and culture. An individualized approach that begins with assessment that includes acknowledging the role of the family caregiver in the trajectory of cancer survivorship is an important first step to inform clinical practice. Family caregivers are unique and their situations and need for support will become evident when they are assessed either during caregiving or during bereavement. Ideally, there is a follow-up provided to family caregivers by known health care providers after the death of the patient to cancer. Listening to their caregiving story is a first step in supporting the caregiver to explore the narrative and constructively find meaning in their experience. Identifying those at most risk of poor outcomes necessitates appropriate referrals to health care and community supports to follow up on emotional and physical health status.

The negative outcomes of grief can be prevented by employing health promotion strategies that also involve the unique needs and strengths of the community, recognizing the sociocultural context such as rural and urban settings and accessibility of services and supports. During caregiving, family caregivers need to be supported in their role through careful assessment and intervention including providing information and support, involving family in a discussion of the goals of care while identifying concerns and questions that can promote a positive caregiver experience (Hudson and Aranda 2013). Without supportive and preventative care focused on the family caregiver, their health is at risk, which can result in even greater demands on an already overburdened health care system.

Nurses, social workers, oncologists, and family practitioners are well positioned to improve current health care approaches, by taking the opportunity to engage in a conversation with a family caregiver, assess their needs and find ways to reduce their suffering. When considering the spectrum of cancer care, the family caregiver is often neglected and taken for granted. What is known about the experience of bereavement for family caregivers is typically underfunded, underinvestigated, and not consistently applied to practice (Hudson 2013). Unheard voices, vulnerable to many deleterious outcomes, are left without systems of support especially once caregiving ends. Paying attention to their needs and prioritizing those at most risk of negative outcomes is an important health promotion strategy that will result in savings to the health care system. By considering the bereaved family caregiver as a cancer survivor, they become part of the spectrum of cancer care as deserving of assessment and intervention to meet their unique needs and support positive outcomes.

References

Agnew, A., Manktelow, R., & Donaghy, K. (2008). User perspective on palliative care services: Experiences of middle-aged partners bereaved through cancer known to social work services in Northern Ireland. *Practice (09503153), 20*(3), 163–180.

Asai, M., Fujimori, M., Akizuki, N., Inagaki, M., Matsui, Y., & Uchitomi, Y. (2010). Psychological states and coping strategies after bereavement among the spouses of cancer patients: A qualitative study. *Psycho-Oncology, 19*(1), 38–45. doi:10.1002/pon.1444

Bowlby, J. (1980). Attachment and loss: Vol. 3. Loss: Sadness and depression. New York: Basic Books.

Canadian Cancer Society's Advisory Committee on Cancer Statistics. (2015). Canadian Cancer Statistics 2015. Retrieved from https://www.cancer.ca/~/media/cancer.ca/CW/cancer%20information/cancer%20101/Canadian%20cancer%20statistics/Canadian-Cancer-Statistics-2015-EN.pdf

Canadian Hospice Palliative Care Association. (2013). A model to guide hospice palliative care. Retrieved from http://www.chpca.net/media/319547/norms-of-practice-eng-web.pdf

Carter, P. A. (2005). Bereaved caregivers' descriptions of sleep: Impact on daily life and the bereavement process. *Oncology Nursing Forum, 32*(4), E70–E75. doi:10.1188/05.ONF.E70-E75

Chan, W. C. H., & Chan, C. L. W. (2011). Acceptance of spousal death: The factor of time in bereaved older adults' search for meaning. *Death Studies, 35*(2), 147–162. doi:10.1080/07481187.2010.535387

Christakis, N. A., & Iwashyna, T. J. (2003). The health impact of health care on families: A matched cohort study of hospice use by decedents and mortality outcomes in surviving, widowed spouses. *Social Science and Medicine, 57*, 465–475.

Clark, P. G., Brethwaite, D. S., & Gnesdiloff, S. (2011). Providing support at time of death from cancer: Results of a 5-year post-bereavement group study. *Journal of social work in end-of-life & palliative care, 7*(2–3), 195–215.

Dean, M., McClement, S., Bond, J. B, Jr., Daeninck, P. J., & Nelson, F. (2005). Parental experiences of adult child death from cancer. *Journal of Palliative Medicine, 8*(4), 751–765.

Dumont, I., Dumont, S., & Mongeau, S. (2008). End-of-life care and the grieving process: Family caregivers who have experienced the loss of a terminal-phase cancer patient. *Qualitative Health Research, 18*(8), 1049–1061.

Ellis, J. (2012). The impact of lung cancer on patients and carers. *Chronic Respiratory Disease, 9* (1), 39–47.
Erlangsen, A., Jeune, B., Bille-Brahe, U., & Vauper, J. W. (2004). Loss of partner and suicide risk among oldest old: A population-based register study. *Age and Ageing, 33*, 378–383. doi:10.1093/ageing/afh128
Grbich, C., Parker, D., & Maddocks, I. (2001). The emotions and coping strategies of caregivers of family members with a terminal cancer. *Journal of Palliative Care, 17*(1), 30–36.
Hegge, M. (1991). A qualitative retrospective study of coping strategies of newly widowed elderly: Effects of anticipatory grieving on the caregiver. *American Journal of Hospice & Palliative Care, 8*(4), 28–34.
Holtslander, L. F., Bally, J. M. G., & Steeves, M. L. (2011). Walking a fine line: An exploration of the experience of finding balance for older persons bereaved after caregiving for a spouse with advanced cancer. *European Journal of Oncology Nursing, 15*(3), 254–259. doi:10.1016/j.ejon.2010.12.004
Holtslander, L., & Duggleby, W. (2008). An inner struggle for hope: Insights from the diaries of bereaved family caregivers. *International Journal of Palliative Nursing, 14*(10), 478–484.
Holtslander, L. F., & Duggleby, W. D. (2009). The hope experience of older bereaved women who cared for a spouse with terminal cancer. *Qualitative Health Research, 19*(3), 388–400. doi:10.1177/1049732308329682
Holtslander, L., & Duggleby, W. (2010). The psychosocial context of bereavement for older women who were caregivers for a spouse with advanced cancer. *Journal of Women & Aging, 22*(2), 109–124. doi:10.1080/08952841003716147
Holtslander, L. F., & McMillan, S. (2011). Depressive symptoms, grief and complicated grief among bereaved family caregivers of advanced cancer patients. *Oncology Nursing Forum, 38*(1), 60–65. doi:10.1188/11.ONF.60-65
Hornjatkevyc, N. L. (2011). With and without: The bereavement experiences of gay men who have lost a partner to non-AIDS-related causes. *Death Studies, 35*(9), 801–823.
Hudson, P. L. (2006). How well do family caregivers cope after caring for a relative with advanced disease and how can health professionals enhance their support? *Journal of Palliative Medicine, 9*(3), 694–703.
Hudson, P. (2013). Improving support for family carers: Key implications for research, policy, and practice. *Palliative Medicine, 27*(7), 581–582. doi:10.1177/0269216313488855
Hudson, P., & Aranda, S. (2013). The Melbourne family support program: Evidence-based strategies that prepare family caregivers for supporting palliative care patients. *BMJ: Supportive and Palliative, 0*, 1 7. doi:10.1136/bmjspcare-2013-000500
Koop, P. M., & Strang, V. R. (2003). The bereavement experience following home-based family caregiving for persons with advanced cancer. *Clinical Nursing Research, 12*(2), 127–144.
Kowalski, S. D., & Bondmass, M. D. (2008). Physiological and psychological symptoms of grief in widows. *Research in Nursing & Health, 31*, 23–30.
Naef, R., Ward, R., Mahrer-Imhof, R., & Grande, G. (2013). Characteristics of the bereavement experience of older persons after spousal loss: An integrative review. *International Journal of Nursing Studies, 50*(8), 1108–1121.
Neimeyer, R. A. (2001). Meaning reconstruction and loss. In R. A. Neimeyer (Ed.), *Meaning reconstruction and the experience of loss* (pp. 1–9). Washington, DC: American Psychological Association.
Neimeyer, R. A., Baldwin, S. A., & Gillies, J. (2006). Continuing bonds and reconstructing meaning: Mitigating complications in bereavement. *Death studies, 30*(8), 715–738.
Pusa, S., Persson, C., & Sundin, K. (2012). Significant others' lived experiences following a lung cancer trajectory: From diagnosis through and after the death of a family member. *European Journal of Oncology Nursing, 16*(1), 34–41. doi:10.1016/j.ejon.2011.02.004
Sandelowski, M., & Barroso, J. (2007). *Handbook for synthesizing qualitative research.* New York: Springer.

Sanderson, C., Lobb, E. A., Mowll, J., Butow, P. N., McGowan, N., & Price, M. A. (2013). Signs of post-traumatic stress disorder in caregivers following an expected death: A qualitative study. *Palliative Medicine, 27*(7), 625–631. doi:10.1177/0269216313483663

Schulz, R., Hebert, R., & Boerner, K. (2008). Bereavement after caregiving. *Geriatrics, 63*(1), 20–22.

Silverman, P. R., & Klass, D. (1996). Introduction: What's the problem? In P. R. Silverman & D. Klass (Eds.), *Continuing bonds: New understandings of grief* (pp. 3–27). Washington, DC: Taylor and Francis.

Stajduhar, K. I., Martin, W., & Cairns, M. (2010). What makes grief difficult? Perspectives from bereaved family caregivers and healthcare providers of advanced cancer patients. *Palliat Support Care, 8*(3), 277–289. doi:10.1017/s1478951510000076

Steeves, R. H. (2002). The rhythms of bereavement. *Family & Community Health, 25*(1), 1–10.

Stroebe, M., Schut, H., & Stroebe, W. (2007). Health outcomes of bereavement. *Lancet, 370*, 1960–1973.

Topf, L., Robinson, C. A., & Bottorff, J. L. (2013). When a desired home death does not occur: The consequences of broken promises. *Journal of Palliative Medicine, 16*(8), 875–880. doi:10.1089/jpm.2012.0541

World Health Organization. (2002). W.H.O. definition of palliative care [Electronic version]. Retrieved February 14, 2005, from http://www.who.int/cancer/palliative/definition/en/

World Health Organization. (2015). Fact sheet on cancer, 2015, from http://www.who.int/mediacentre/factsheets/fs297/en/

Index

A
Acculturation, 2
  definition, 37
  Latinos, 26
  Latvians, 37, 38
  Mexican Americans, 39
  Muslims, 60
Acute lymphoblastic leukemia (ALL), 114
Acute myelogenous leukemia (AML), 114
Adenocarcinoma, 129
Adolescent and young adult (AYA), 71, 74
  cancer care programming, 88
  implications and future research, 87
Adolescent resilience model (ARM), 3, 32
Adult cancers, 113–114
Aging
  and culture, 2–3
  and ethnicity, 2
  population, 143, 144, 151
Art therapy (art-making), women with breast cancer
  on artist's book format, 78
  benefits, 71
  demographic data and disease characteristics, 75–76
  inclusion criteria, 74
  intervention, 74–75
  and meaning-making process, 72
  narrative-based interviews
    connections, 84–87
    on their own terms, 82–84
    two selves, 80–82
    unspeakable losses and challenging stereotypes, 78–80
  narrative inquiry, 77
  in oncology, 71
  qualitative analysis, 77
  qualitative inquiry, 76
  quality of life, 75
  setting, 73
  study design, 72–73
  subjects/patients and recruitment, 73
Assimilation theory, 2, 26
Association of Oncology Social Workers, 134
Attachment theory, 150

B
Bereaved caregivers, 150–151
  assessment, 148
  clinical practice, 151–152
  family caregivers, 144–145
  lack of support, 147
  mental health issues, 146–147
  metasynthesis of qualitative research
    goal, 145
    overwhelming and unpredictable emotions, 146
    research and practice source, 145
  overall morbidity and mortality, 144
  supporting and valuing, 149–150
Biopsychosocial model, 69
Breast cancer
  demographic information, 101
  immigrant population of, 37, 51
  Latino cancer survivors, *see* Latino cancer survivors
  Muslim women with, *see* Muslim women with breast cancer
  quality of life of young adult, *see* Art therapy (art-making), women with breast cancer
  study, 94, 96, 98

C
Canadian Association of Psychosocial Oncology (CAPO), 11
Canadian Breast Cancer Foundation, 68
Canadian Cancer Society, 67, 70, 144

T.R. Fitzpatrick (ed.), *Treating Vulnerable Populations of Cancer Survivors: A Biopsychosocial Approach*, DOI 10.1007/978-3-319-32364-0

Canadian Hospice Palliative Care Association (CHPCA), 143, 145
Canadian Hospital Accreditation Board for Regional Cancer Centers, 8
Canadian problem checklist, 11
Cancer. *See also* Breast cancer
  aging, 2
  and emotional health, 38
  ethnicity, 2
  experience and supportive interventions of Latvian immigrants, *see* Latvian immigrants, cancer experience and supportive interventions
  family and community support, 39
  history, 7
  and immigrants, 38
  in Latvians, 38–39
  rehabilitation and survivorship care, 7
  stress and coping mechanism, 1–2
Cancer survivors
  adolescents and young adults (AYAs), 74
  children and adolescent, theoretical perspectives, 3–4
  Latvian immigrants, cancer experience and supportive interventions
    cultural and ethnic ties, 46
    first generation immigrants, 42–43
    personal account, 44
    traditional medical interventions, 48
  young children, 25
Cancer survivors from community-based cancer support program, 106
  control variables, 100–101
  correlation matrix, 103
  data analysis, 101
  data collection, 98–99
  demographic data, 101–102
  direct effect model, 97
  fear of recurrence, 105
    clinical practice, 106
    dependent variable, 99–100
    factors, 94
    hypothesis, 97
    and LOC, 95–96
    patient outcomes, 95
    and physical activity, 96
    prevalence, 94
    regression analyses, 103, 104
    theoretical perspectives, 96
  future research, 107
  limitations, 107
  LOC and physical activity, 105
    clinical practice, 106
    and fear of recurrence, 95–96
    hypothesis, 98
    independent variable, 100
    regression analyses, 103–104
    relationship between, 93, 105
    theoretical perspectives, 97
  sample, 98
  site and data, 98
Cancer survivorship, 8, 10, 59, 105, 112, 119, 144, 151
Cancer Wellness Centre, 73
Chemotherapy, 23, 25, 28, 62, 73, 100, 114–117, 129, 136–139
Childhood cancers. *See* Pediatric cancer
Clear-cell sarcoma, 114
Complementary and alternative medicine (CAM), 68, 70–71
Complexity paradigm, 27
Coping, 48, 49, 51, 62, 69, 82, 95–97, 105, 106
  booklet on, 12–14
  definition, 2
  efficacy, 10
  LOC and physical activity and, 103–104
  mechanism, 1–2
  strategies, 39, 99, 101, 134, 138, 148
Cultural pluralism, 2, 26
Culture and social class model, 4

D

Dehydration, 115
Demographic information, 24, 30, 57, 67–68, 75–76, 101–102, 127
Dental caries (dental decay), 113, 115, 116
Dental infections, 115
Depression, 8–10, 31, 38, 58, 69, 95, 133, 134, 144, 147
Direct effect model, 96–98, 101, 105, 106
Distress screening, Canada
  Canadian problem list, 16–18
  intervention
    booklet on coping, 12–14
    Canadian problem checklist, 11
    coping efficacy, 10
    distress thermometer, 11
    ESAS, 10–11
    psychosocial educational, 8
  levels, 16
  management, 14–15
  prevention, 8
  recommendations, 16–20
  self-care strategies, 9
  time requirement, 18
  total care person-centered cancer system, 8
Distress thermometer
  outcomes, 20

stress, measure and management of, 11
Double jeopardy hypothesis, 2
Dysphagia, 129, 133, 136, 137, 139

E
Eastern Cooperative Oncology Group (ECOG) Performance Status, 138
Edmonton Symptom Assessment Scale (ESAS), 10–11
Endoscopic resection, 129
Esophageal cancer survivors
causes, 129
epidemiology and demographics, 127
future perspectives, 128–139
incidence rates, 128
men *vs.* women patients, 128
prognosis, 129
quality of life
HRQoL, 130–132
multidimensional concept, 130
risk factors, 128
squamous cell carcinoma, 129
therapeutic interventions
nursing and physician, 138
nutrition, 135–138
psychosocial problems, 133–134
social support, 132–133
social worker and oncologists, 134–135
treatment, 129
Esophagus, anatomical features, 128
Ethnicity, 2, 25, 51
European Organization for the Research and Treatment of Cancer (EORTC), 131

F
Family caregivers, 150
as cancer survivorship, 143–144
clinical practice, implications for, 151–152
health care system, 143
as "secondary survivor", 144
Fatalismo (coping), 32
Fear of cancer recurrence inventory (FCRI), 99
Fear of recurrence, cancer survivors, 105
clinical practice, 106
definition, 93
dependent variable, 99–100
factors, 94
hypothesis, 97
and LOC, 95–96
patient outcomes, 95
and physical activity, 96
prevalence, 94
regression analyses, 103, 104
theoretical perspectives, 96
Functional Assessment of Cancer Therapy (FACT), 131

G
Germ cell tumors, 114
Gliomas, 114

H
Halal food, 62
Health Related Quality of Life (HRQoL), 130
Hematopoietic stem cell transplantation (HSCT), 115
Hepatoblastoma, 114
Hodgkin's lymphoma, 114
Hope and locus of control, concept of, 3
Hope & Cope Wellness Centre, 88
Hypodontia, 116

I
Institutional Review Board (IRB), 73
International Association for Dental Research and International Society of Pediatric Oncology, 117
Internet-based information, 9

L
Laparoscopic resection, 129
Latino cancer survivors, 30–31
age and cultural interventions
church-based interventions, 30
educational intervention, 30
focus groups, 29
physical activities, 27–28
senior centers, 29
support groups, 28–29
in children and adolescence
cancer experience, 26–27
clinical practice, 31–33
factors, 23
quality of life, 25
statistics, 25
demographic information, 24
theoretical perspectives, 25–26
Latvian immigrants, cancer experience and supportive interventions, 50–51
cancer caregivers
collusion and coping forms, 48–49
first generation and first immigrants, 43
language and community supports, 46–47
limited care, 44–45
cancer preventative behaviors, 51
cancer survivors
cultural and ethnic ties, 46

first generation immigrants, 42–43
personal account, 44
traditional medical interventions, 48
clinical practice, 51–52
data, 40
data collection procedures, 40
data recording, 42
healthcare providers, 43, 45, 47, 49
interview protocol, 40–42
qualitative research design and approach, 39
sample, 40, 41
spiritual caregivers
different roles, 45–46
diversity of treatments and coping skills, 49–50
examples, 44
private and community experience, 47
Leukemia, 31, 114, 116
Loneliness, 25, 27, 32, 51, 59, 144, 146, 147, 151
Loss of control (LOC), cancer survivors, 105
clinical practice, 106
definition, 93
and fear of recurrence, 95–96
hypothesis, 98
independent variable, 100
regression analyses, 103–104
relationship between, 93, 105
theoretical perspectives, 97
Loss of normal childhood, 25, 27
Lymphomas, 114

M

Mammogram, 24, 30, 44, 139
Mammography, 57, 60, 62
Mastery, concept of, 2
Meaning-making process, 72, 77, 78, 149, 150
Medicaid fee-for-service program, 30
Meditation, 14, 48, 50, 61, 68
Metabolic equivalency tasks (METs), 100, 101, 103, 107
Metastatic cancer, 68
Microdontia, 116
Modernization theory, 2, 25
Mouth infections, 115
Multimodal therapy, 129
Muslim women with breast cancer
cross-cultural curative factors, 62–63
diverse population, 63
fear and relapse, 59
health challenges, 58
health disparities
and cancer demographics, 57
and survivorship, 57–58
implications for treatment, 61–62
religion-related factors, 60–61
social support, 59
spiritual dimension, requirement of, 59
theoretical perspectives, 61
in United States, 56, 59–60

N

National Cancer Institute (NCI), 8, 112, 129
National Institute of Dental and Craniofacial Research, 119
Neuman's step-by-step approach, 77, 78
Non-Hodgkin's lymphoma, 114
Nueva Luz, 30

O

Oral health issues, pediatric cancer survivors. *See* Pediatric cancer
Oral mucositis, 115, 118, 120

P

Pan Canadian Practice Guidelines, 11
Pap test screening, 95
Pediatric cancer
vs. adult cancers, 113–114
cancer therapy effects, 113
clear-cell sarcoma, 114
germ cell tumors, 114
gliomas, 114
leukemias, 114
lymphomas, 114
in North America, 111
oral side-effects, 111
PRISMA flow diagram, 122
QOL, *see* Quality of life (QOL)
retinoblastoma, 114
sarcomas, 114
scoping review study, 117
survival rates, 111
treatment and its effect on oral health
early oral effects, 114, 115
late oral effects and QOL, 114–116
Wilm's tumor, 114
Peristalsis, 128
Personalisma, 26
Physical activity, cancer survivors, 105
clinical practice, 106
definition, 93–94
and fear of recurrence, 96
hypothesis, 98
independent variable, 100
regression analyses, 103–104
relationship between, 93, 105

theoretical perspectives, 97
Posttraumatic stress disorder (PTSD), 3
Promotora Intervention, The, 30
Psychological distress, 37, 99
Psycho-oncology, 7
Psychosocial distress, 115

Q
Quality of life (QOL), 10
cancer-related, 1
definition, 1, 24
esophageal cancer survivors
HRQoL, 130–132
multidimensional concept, 130
pediatric cancer patient, 111, 120, 121
assessments, 113
defined, 112
management, 117–118
multidimensional concept, 112
multi-disciplinary approach, 119
physical domain, 118
psychological and social domains, 118
studies, 112
women with breast cancer, 75
Quality of Life Questionnaire-Core 30 (QLQ-C30), 131

R
Radiation therapy, 73, 113, 115, 116
Radiotherapy
esophagus cancer, 129, 136
pediatric cancers, 114, 116, 117
Reiki, 68
Resilience model, 3–4
Resting metabolic rate (RMR), 107
Retinoblastoma, 114
Rhabdomyosarcoma, 114
Root stunting, 116

S
Sarcomas, 114
Self-efficacy, 2, 9, 10
Shari'a law, 60
Social isolation, 25, 27, 32, 147
SPSS 11.01 statistical software program, 101
Squamous cell carcinoma, 129
Stem cell transplantation, 114
Strength-based perspective, 3
Suicide, 69, 133, 144, 147
Survivorship care plans, 9, 58, 63
Symbolic interactionsim, 26

T
Taste disturbances, 115
Theoretical perspectives
art therapy, 71
culture and social class model, 4
double jeopardy, 25
fear of recurrence, 96–97
locus of control, 96–97
modernization theory, 25
Muslim women with breast cancer, 61
post-traumatic stress disorder, 3
resilience model, 3–4
strength-based perspective, 3
stress and coping model, 1–2
Therapeutic interventions
art therapy, 74–75
caregivers, 43–50
church-based interventions, 30
clinical trials, 121
community cancer support centers, 30
community services, 41
coping resources, 3, 10, 12–14
dental health, 112, 120–121
educational resources, 10, 24, 30
family caregiving, 149–150
fear of recurrence, 106
household activities, 24, 27, 94
leisure activities, 24, 27, 94
nursing and physician, 138
nutrition, 135–138
physical activity and LOC, 106
psychosocial problems, 133–134
senior centers, 29
social support, 132–133
social worker and oncologists, 134–135
support groups, 24, 28–29, 134, 138
Trismus, 116

U
United States
breast cancer
Muslim women, *see* Muslim women with breast cancer
prevalence, 55
survivorship, 55–56
Institutes of Medicine (IOM), 8

W
Wilm's tumor, 114
Women with breast cancer
art therapy (art-making)

on artist's book format, 78
benefits, 71
demographic data and disease characteristics, 75–76
inclusion criteria, 74
intervention, 74–75
and meaning-making process, 72
narrative-based interviews, 78–87
narrative inquiry, 77
in oncology, 71
qualitative analysis, 77
qualitative inquiry, 76
setting, 73
study design, 72–73
subjects/patients and recruitment, 73
CAM, 70–71
diagnosis, 68
fertility and childrearing, 69–70
risk of depression, 69
support group for, 68

X

Xerostomia (dry mouth), 115

Y

Yoga, 68
Young adult art therapy programming, 88

CPSIA information can be obtained
at www.ICGtesting.com
Printed in the USA
LVOW05*2045060717
540475LV00008B/188/P

9 783319 323626